What to Know

Improving Your Health

It has often been said that it's difficult to appreciate all that life offers without good health. Yet when it comes to dealing with health issues, or simply improving already good health, the way is not always very clear. Especially for those interested in approaches other than the traditional Western medical route, the options can be daunting and confusing.

Keys to a Vibrantly Healthy, Long Life lays out a clear path for dealing with health and vitality. While it centers around Debra Gaffney's substantial experience as an Acupuncture Physician, it goes far beyond that one approach because Debra's practice encompasses a wide range of healing modalities. Among the topics covered are:

- Acupuncture – from needling and related practices such as cupping, gua sha and moxibustion to leading edge discoveries in electro-acupuncture

- Nutrition – including explanations of food components, elements of Oriental nutrition, the value of supplements, and ailment-specific foods

- Herbal medicine – the hows and whys

- Homeopathics – what they are and how they work

- Allopathic (prescription) drugs and their place in healing

- Lifestyle products – shampoo, toothpaste, cosmetics

- Stretching, prayer & meditation, breathing

There is also a section containing an extensive list of physical ailments, from allergies to thyroid conditions, and how they have been successfully addressed with acupuncture.

Debra puts it all into context, explaining how many different approaches might be included in an overall health plan. She describes how her practice integrates a range of modalities so you have a sense of what you might look for when evaluating a practitioner's approach.

The book covers a lot of ground, and goes satisfyingly deep in its explorations. It is information-rich and well grounded in science as well as experience. It is an easy-to-use reference that is a valuable addition to any health library.

About the Author

Debra Gaffney, A.P., C.C.P.A., is a healer in the true sense of the word. Her foundation is in Oriental medicine, including acupuncture and herbology. Upon that base she built a healing practice that incorporates her extensive experience with nutrition, homeopathy, and other 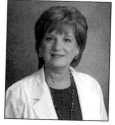 natural health-supporting approaches. In 2002 she developed a method for neutralizing food and environmental sensitivities called AcuSET(SM) that has restored thousands of her patients to full lives of health and happiness.

Among her many degrees and certifications, Debra is a Diplomate in Acupuncture and Oriental Medicine and a certified Chiropractic Physician Assistant.

Debra is relentless in her pursuit of knowledge in health and the healing arts, frequently taking classes and workshops to expand her ability to help others. She also enjoys regular participation in Jazzercise, Tai Chi and Yoga. Debra lives with her husband, Dr. John Gaffney, a Chiropractic Physician, in DeLand, Florida, where she practices, writes, and enjoys playing with their two dogs and two cats.

Keys to a
Vibrantly Healthy, Long Life

Keys to a
Vibrantly Healthy, Long Life

Insights and Information on Healing, Health and Well-Being

Debra Gaffney, A.P., C.C.P.A.
Acupuncture Physician

SERENITY PASS PRESS
DELAND, FLORIDA

Printed in the United States of America

Publisher's Cataloguing-in-Publication

Gaffney, Debra P.

    Keys to a vibrantly healthy, long life : insights and information on healing, health and well-being / Debra Gaffney. -- Deland, Fla. : Serenity Pass Press, c2011.

      p. ; cm.

      ISBN: 978-0-615-42602-0
      Includes index.

      1. Holistic medicine. 2. Alternative medicine. 3. Acupuncture. 4. Nutrition. 5. Self-care, Health. I. Title.

R733 .G34 2011   2010942747
615.5--dc22   1101

Book Consultant: Ellen Reid
Book Cover& Interior Design: Ghislain Viau

To the Reader

The field of acupuncture and the treatment of allergies and sensitivities and nutrition are constantly changing. The author has taken great care in writing truthfully her understanding of the above health care modalities. The author always recommends her patients keep open lines of communication with their other health care practitioners. At no time does the author recommend her patients quit taking their prescription drugs without the knowledge of their prescribing doctors.

This publication is designed to educate and provide general information regarding the subject matter covered. It is not intended to replace the counsel of other professional advisors. The reader is encouraged to consult with his or her own advisors regarding specific situations. While the author has taken reasonable precautions in the preparation of this book and believes the facts presented within the book are accurate, neither the publisher nor author assumes any responsibility for errors or omissions. The author and publisher specifically disclaim any liability resulting from the use or application of the information contained in this book. The information within this book is not intended to serve as emotional or therapeutic advice related to individual situations.

Contents

Acknowledgments

This is my second book, and again I thank my wonderful husband, number-one mentor, and biggest supporter, John Gaffney, D.C. He helped me with research for this book, saw more in me than I ever did, and pushed me to achieve the confidence to dedicate my life to helping sick people regain their health.

I'm grateful to Ellen Reid, the best book shepherd, and her wonderfully patient team members who brought this book together. It was fun having "people" to guide and assist in making this book make sense! What amazing work they do!

I extend my gratitude to Denise Heist for teaching me how to use the computer, for re-typing my manuscript again, and for finding the correct spelling for all those "strange words." I also thank a new member of my book team—Joanne Milleson. Joanne taught me how to utilize my new computer setup in ways I didn't know existed. Joanne's patience is unfathomable.

I also thank Cheryl Floyd, owner and publisher of *Natural Awakenings Magazine* and a professional storyteller; she kept me laughing and ignited my creativity!

I express my thanks to Buffy Williams for her encouragement, e-mails, and beautiful affirmations; Jonathan Ellis for support during this process; Reverend Nancy Saputro for keeping me on the right track; Dr. Denis Gulliver for acting as a sounding board and providing encouragement; Christine Conforti, my dear friend of thirty years, for her active listening; and Cristal, my Jazzercise instructor, who enabled me to Jazzercise as a "treat" for hours of writing (Cristal has no idea of the wonderful effect she has on people)!

Of course, I also thank my mom and dad, Elizabeth and Jim Pardee, my sister Michele, my brother Jim, Aunt Eileen, and Uncle Tom for their support and encouragement. I especially thank Uncle Jack for taking my husband on vacation for five days so I could write. Thanks to Aunt Jane and Uncle Bart for housing them and entertaining them with my cousins William and Matthew.

Most of all, I thank my patients. Thousands of them participated in the case histories, testimonials, and referrals. They had faith in me and followed my suggestions and kept my spirits up while we worked on their problems.

Lastly, I thank my staff members, who are always constant in their support, especially Christina, Rose Mary and Nancy. They help keep me balanced and see the humor in the difficult situations we face regularly. Laughter really is the best medicine.

I wrote this book as an aid for my patients but it can be of help to anyone interested in learning a "take charge" healthy way of living. Anyone can read this book and garner an understanding of acupuncture and alternative health care. I hope you share this information with your family, friends, and medical doctors. You might find it hard to believe some of the things you read in this book. Every day my staff and I witness amazing results.

I've included a few patient testimonials in this book. My patients have enjoyed reading them through the years and have told me the testimonials have encouraged them to try specific techniques.

I've spent most of my life studying nutrition, acupuncture, and chiropractic. Indeed, a picture shows me at age four reading a book on nutrition—the book's upside down, but I'm still reading it. I was the kid that climbed to the top cabinet to get a bottle of Brewer's Yeast at age two. I remember eating liver and spinach as a child and loving it. I also remember telling Mom I could feel the vitamins marching in my mouth.

I have put my heart, soul, blood, sweat, tears, and Qi in this book and in my practice. It distresses me to see people of any age suffer needlessly. If you're not sure that we or acupuncture can help you, I beg you to ask us or call your local Acupuncture Physician. Eighty-five percent of my patients have been helped and are satisfied. I continue to try to find a way to help the remaining 15 percent who weren't completely satisfied. There are no guarantees in life or medicine, but acupuncture cannot hurt you in any way. The only side effects are healthy, wonderful side effects—more energy, a general sense of well-being, and an end to sneezing, runny noses, joint pains, rashes, headaches, and bowel problems.

You don't have to die prematurely from disease; there's another way! You can live a long healthy life and then pass simply because you are very old and your body finally wears out after serving you well for many, many years. Remember when we were kids and people died merely from old age? That's how I plan to go! But what about you?

My typical patient is a woman between forty and seventy years old. She has suffered for years with a myriad of problems, takes four to six medications a day, and can't remember the last time she felt good. She is usually overweight, which baffles her. She wakes up planning her next nap. She works and has a family. My office is her last resort. In the past, men visited us only when their wives were tired of their snoring or lack of energy. However, I am seeing a change in this in the last three years. Men don't want to end up sick and on lots of medications like their parents or grandparents either.

In the last thirty years, medicine has transformed dramatically in our country. When I was in grade school, only one child in my class was overweight. One had asthma and one had allergies. We never heard the phrases "learning disabled" or ADD. We ate bagged lunches from home and played outside. We rarely went to a doctor. We went to bed at night and slept all night. We never ate in fast-food restaurants. We were healthy and happy.

Now, I talk to teachers who tell me children are always missing school because of illness or attending school sick, which spreads the "sickness." The school nurse hands out medicine prescribed by doctors. I see children in my office who have been sick since they were born. Their moms always say the same thing: "When you get him/her better, I'll come to see you for the allergies I've had since childhood. Could I have passed this on to my children?"

Chapter I

History of Acupuncture

Over five thousand years ago, Chinese doctors tried to find better ways to treat their patients. These observant doctors had little to work with, so they would study their patients by examining the color of their skin and eyes as well as their teeth, gums, and tongue. The doctor would also touch the patients, feeling the muscles for tightness, looseness, lumps, heat, and cold.

Answers to specific questions provided information about every aspect of the patient's lifestyle. Were cool days enjoyable, or did the patient huddle by the fire? When it rained, did the patient feel his aches more? What happened when it was windy? What did her bowel movements, urine, vomit, and so on look like? Did heat feel better or did it make the patient uncomfortable? What food did he enjoy eating and which foods made him sick? Nothing was left unasked.

At the regional gatherings, the doctors would compare notes. Symptoms were categorized; conditions were examined. Did the patients in the southern part experience the same conditions as patients in the north? The patient who had fallen off a roof would tell his doctor whether it felt better or worse when his wife rubbed his back. Some doctors tried using a flat stone and pressing down on the patient's spine. It felt good; in fact, if the stone was heated, it felt even better. The doctors also discussed what worked and didn't work in herbal medicines. Health care did not "just happen" but was experimented with for thousands of years.

Fast-forward to a few thousand years later, approximately 2000 BC, and doctors still gathered to learn from each other about techniques and instruments. Prisoners and family members of the doctors endured experiments. "Lines" could be traced along the body where tightness would be felt. Doctors began using bamboo and bone rather than stone for needles; these needles would actually go into the sore spots and relieve pain. When these new needles were inserted, sometimes the pain would go away. If not, then other "points" or "lines" were used. In 1760 BC during the Shang Dynasty, bronze was used in manufacturing needles; gold and silver came about in 500 BC; and in 200 BC, steel was created.

Sometime between 300 and 100 BC, Ch'I Po wrote *The Huang Di Nei Ching Su Wen*, a book that contained detailed descriptions of pathology, treatment plans, anatomy, and physiology. It talked about Yin and Yang and described organs and diseases of the body. The Nei Ching talked about 160 points for needling the body to foster healing. It described different needling techniques and nine different needles. Translations of this book are still studied today.

During the sixteenth century, the physician Li Shi Shen wrote fifty volumes of a book called *Ben Cao Gang Nu* (Material Medica). The text discussed uses for over 1,500 herbs and contained 10,000 herbal prescriptions. Li Shi Shen also established the pulse positions acupuncturists still use today. As the benefits of acupuncture spread, several other countries, including Japan, Korea, India, and Pakistan began using acupuncture techniques.

Acupuncture arrived in the United States with the migration of the Chinese in the nineteenth century. Patients adventurous enough to see a practitioner in San Francisco at that time would have been examined and treated in almost the same way that patients are examined and treated today. Why mess with something that works? After centuries of use, acupuncture has proven that it helps the body heal itself. Acupuncture treats the body as a whole and not a conglomeration of disconnected body parts.

Acupuncture enjoyed an earlier and more visible exposure in Europe than in America. A Dutch doctor, W. Ten Rhyne (or Willem Ten Rhijne as he is referenced in some sources) studied in Japan where a Dutch company employed him. Drawing upon his discoveries in Japan, in 1683, Rhyne wrote the earliest published European report on acupuncture.

After visiting China and upon their return to France in 1735, a group of Jesuit priests wrote about acupuncture and the Chinese method of diagnosing. Strikingly, I still employ one technique that is referenced in their books. In the nineteenth century, European doctors (particularly in England, Germany, and Italy) used acupuncture to treat patients suffering from neuralgia and rheumatism.

After the late nineteenth century, most European doctors did not practice Asian medicine, but instead used needles to explore tumors or for local pain relief. Medicine changed rapidly, and homeopathy (which has its roots much earlier in the 1700s) was in vogue.

Doctors did not implement acupuncture in Europe again until the 1950s. At that time, acupuncture spread across Europe and even the Middle East. Accordingly, most of the acupuncture research outside of Asia was performed in France and Germany.

U.S. interest in acupuncture sparked in 1972 while President Nixon traveled to China. One of the reporters covering the trip, James Reston, suffered an appendicitis attack. After surgery, doctors administered acupuncture to control his pain. Reston wrote about his experience in *The New York Times*. American doctors grew fascinated by acupuncture and started hiring doctors from China or traveling to China to learn for themselves.

In the last ten years, the United States has increasingly conducted more research. Acupuncture information and research is available in most teaching hospitals such as Shands at the University of Florida in Gainesville and all the Mayo clinics. The National Institutes of Health (NIH) is conducting approximately seventy different acupuncture studies. One of my Asian teachers asked why the American people would not accept acupuncture until they researched it for years when Asia had performed over five thousand years of constant research. A good "point"!

In a 2007 survey, 3.2 million Americans had received acupuncture. In 2001 that figure was 2.1 million. Today, you can't pick up a magazine without reading an article on acupuncture. Additionally, acupuncture appears on the television almost weekly. Even Oprah tried it on live TV, backed by Dr. Oz, a large acupuncturist supporter as well.

Why is acupuncture popular in the United States now? Well, most people sense that there must be a better way to achieve and maintain health. After all, their parents and grandparents did just fine and rarely took pills or saw a doctor. Why are we so sickly and dependent on drugs when we live with a plethora of technology that ensures healthy food, water, and air? Why do we not know how to get healthy and stay that way?

People are tired of a health care system that does not look at them as people but as hearts, lungs, or joints—and diseased ones at that, without any hope for health. People are tired of taking pills that cause other problems and send them to yet another doctor for more pills. Acupuncture is popular in the United States because it works.

Chapter 2

What Is Acupuncture and Oriental Medicine?

Sometimes, explaining acupuncture is easy, and other days, it's not. Records and books prove that Asian and Indian doctors implemented acupuncture over 4000 years ago. Acupuncture Physicians use thousands-of-years-old formulas and acupoints that still work. We can now also document the results.

For a simple definition, acupuncture is a modality that involves gently inserting very fine needles into the skin in a shallow depth, while Oriental Medicine (OM) is the description of a modality that implements diagnosis techniques and needles, herbs, Gua Sha, and moxa to treat health problems.

The following pages will hopefully leave you with a better understanding of a healthcare system that dates back to the times when the pyramids were under construction. If a system works and lasts this long, there has to be value to it. In contrast, note that some procedures and allopathic medicines are taken off the market every year.

The Latest Research

I can always sense people's surprise when I tell them of acupuncture trials and studies in the United States. We are years behind in research compared to Europe, but we are making progress. It's easy to find the latest studies—just visit www.Acufinder.com and go to the learning center. Over seventy studies and trials have recently been conducted across the country according to my sources. Let me list some of the most current and interesting trials below:

- In 2005, Oregon Health and Science University found acupuncture to be effective in the treatment of bladder control.

- Harvard Medical School tested thirteen volunteers by using MRI scanners. They inserted a needle at the Large Intestine 4 on the hand and manipulated the needle. This increased signal intensity in a key region of the brain. Researchers concluded acupuncture regulates multiple physiological systems.

- A study conducted in Taiwan and published in *The American Journal of Physiology* pointed to the effectiveness of Electro-Acupuncture in reducing the key mechanism of GERD.

- A 2006 survey of the American Hospital Association revealed more than one in four hospitals in the U.S. offered alternative therapies including acupuncture (39%). This service was more than likely paid out of the patient's pocket.

- In 2007, a double blind study at the Mayo Clinic found acupuncture was helpful in treating fatigue and anxiety in fibromyalgia patients.

- The American College of Chest Physicians recommended acupuncture for lung cancer patients for fatigue, dyspena, chemo-induced neuropathy, anxiety, nausea, and vomiting.

- A new study published in *The Journal of Clinical Oncology* reported that acupuncture may be an effective method for treating joint problems caused by medications for breast cancer patients.

- Research from Duke University in 2007 concluded that acupuncture before and after surgery reduced the levels of postoperative pain and decreased the dosage of needed pain killers.

- A study in 2005 showed reduced rates of nausea, itchiness, and dizziness with acupuncture.

- In the *British Medical Journal's* February 2008 edition, trials involving 1,366 women showed a success rate of 65 percent of IVF (In Vitro Fertilization) after acupuncture. This research was carried out at the University of Maryland in the United States and Amsterdam.

- A very interesting use of acupuncture was utilized in Iraq. Researchers administered acupuncture to successfully perform 200 cesarean births due to shortages of drugs. Post-surgery, 45 percent of the women did not require the drug commonly administered to stimulate womb contractions for healing.

- In November 2008, Harvard Medical School published evidence showing endogenous opiods (internal natural pain-relieving chemicals) as central to the experience of pain and acupuncture analgesia. They found signal changes in the brain that reduced pain with the use of acupuncture.

- In 2007, research studied the effectiveness of acupuncture on Post Traumatic Stress Disorder, which can be caused from any trauma, natural disaster, accident, or military combat. The study involved seventy-three people and was supported by the NIH and the National Center for Complementary and Alternative Medicine. Acupuncture proved viable for the treatment of PTSD in some participants, who even stated they felt they were significantly helped.

- The March 2008 edition of *Headache* confirmed that acupuncture reduces migraines and works better than drugs alone. I have had personal success with relieving my patients of headaches and migraines.

- In September 2008, *Cephalalgia* showed acupuncture reduces the severity of headaches and chronic migraines. The German study followed 15,000 adults.

- The newest excitement came this past month (August 2010). The New England School of Acupuncture is the recipient of a 1.2 million dollar, U.S. Department of Defense grant to fund clinical trials on acupuncture's effectiveness on the Gulf War illness.

- In May 2010, *Nature Neuroscience* stated that a neuro-modulator called adenosine A1 receptor is released during acupuncture, which may be the reason why acupuncture can relieve pain.

Principles

Tong bing yi zhi
Yi bing ting zhi
(The same disease, different treatments
Different disease, the same treatment)

This ancient Chinese saying explains the basis of Oriental Medicine. Each person is entirely different from every other person. To diagnose and treat patients in Oriental medicine, we use different ideas and procedures. With balance and harmony in the body and mind comes health. When the balance is upset, then people become sick. This imbalance can take days, months, or years to accumulate, but they will get sick unless harmony and balance are restored.

Five Elements

Five-element acupuncture involves two similar treatments and systems of diagnosing. The one treatment most often implemented by acupuncture physicians is the Chinese form. In Chinese five-element acupuncture, each meridian has its own time of day, color, odor, sound, emotion, flavor, and season. We can attach a Meridian Complex to each patient to further narrow down the treatment plan. We look at your color (red, green, yellow, white, or blue). These colors are shown around your eyes, cheeks, and around your mouth. We listen to your voice, while you're singing, crying, laughing, groaning, or shouting. These sounds vary in degrees; we don't honestly get patients that shout in the clinic.

There are different odors for each meridian. Usually after five minutes, I have you pinpointed to (at the most) two meridians. People tend to have most of their health problems in three meridians. We then proceed to put together a treatment protocol with all of this in mind. The other method is called Worsley Five Element Acupuncture. This procedure takes the above information to another level and is very precise in diagnosing and treating. My interpretation is they may only treat Acupoints on the meridian that is "yours." I liken it to your "sign" in acupuncture.

Patterns

Practitioners look at eight parameters first. Is the patient hot or cold? Is the injured area hot, cold, or somewhere in between? If it is a Cold condition, it can present as cramps, pain, or spasms. Are the stools watery? Are there large amounts of pale urine? Is the phlegm white, clear, or watery? If it is a Hot condition, the tongue can be dry and red. The urine can be dark and be produced in smaller amounts of it. Phlegm can be yellow or green. There can be rashes. Is it an exterior or surface condition, the common cold, something in the interior or deeper (feels better to rub it or to put pressure on it)? Is it a Yin or Yang condition? We decide if it is a Dry (hacking cough, constipation) or Damp condition (limbs feel heavy, sluggish feeling, head feels swollen and tight). This is just one way we look at our patients and some of the questions we ask.

Hoary Treatments

Each meridian has its own time of day and time of year (among other things). If a patient arrives between three and five on a wintery evening with bladder problems—and I give them an acupuncture treatment—this is a Hoary treatment. I always keep in mind the time of day that they come in and schedule treatments for that specific meridian's time, especially if it is the season for that problem or meridian.

I like to treat the corresponding meridians in the season. For example, I have my patients come in for treatments four times a year. I call it the Fire Meridian Prevention treatment if it is in June or July or a Water treatment for the Kidney and Bladder Meridian. The ancient acupuncturists recommended that patients receive treatment four times a year or every season change. Different health problems arise up at different seasons (for example, sinus in the spring or fall).

Sedation vs. Tonification

Patients always inquire about the length of the treatments. Some want long sessions and some can barely lie still for fifteen minutes. The general rule is the shorter the treatment, the more tonifying and the longer the more sedating. If there is pain, heat, and swelling, we may treat that patient longer than someone in a weakened condition (for example, after the flu). The acupuncture physician must make many decisions to determine the appropriate treatment. Some patients may need acupuncture on the front of the body, hands, legs, and feet; or perhaps the patient needs a treatment on the back, which will take more time. Years of studying, class work, and experience help the acupuncturist make an informed decisions.

Auriculotherapy (Ear Acupuncture)

Each ear has over 160 points that correspond to body parts and systems. There is truly a complete body map in each ear. A procedure called auriculotherapy involves the shallow insertion of tiny needles into the external ear. I have always felt that using this procedure created a more thorough treatment. I use the incredible calming points on the ear during every treatment. Some acupuncture physicians don't use the ear as part of the treatment, some focus solely on the ears, and others like me facilitate all parts of the body. I always feel acupuncture on the ears is very relaxing, although I honor the request of some patients that do not like their ears touched.

Meridians

An easy way to understand acupuncture and Oriental medicine is to visualize your body as a Christmas tree with fourteen strands of lights. Some of your light bulbs are blinking nicely. Some are blinking fast; some are only dully lit; and some aren't blinking at all. These light bulbs are your acupuncture points.

The electrical wires for the strand of lights are the meridians (pathways/channels) and the current running through the "wires" is Qi (energy). The meridians all have a color, odor, sound, emotion (way of being), pulse, flavor, time of day, and season. The meridians are translated into English and named after organ systems. The meridians are the Lung, Large Intestine, Stomach, Spleen, Heart, Small Intestine, Bladder, Kidney, Pericardium, Triple Warmer, Gallbladder, and Liver. Meridians work with more than the organs named. For example, the Lung Meridian deals with respiratory tissues and skin; the Large Intestine Meridian works with the large intestines, throat, and sinus. The emotions involved with those two meridians are letting go, grief, and sorrow. The color is white; the time of day is three AM to seven AM, and the season is fall.

The Kidney Meridian handles problems with the kidneys, hair, teeth, joints, memory, reproduction system, spine, brain, feet, and many other bodily functions. The Bladder Meridian works with the bladder and urine, and the acupoints for the Bladder Meridian start by the eyes, go up the head, down the spine, and down the back of the leg to the little toe. Associated with this meridian, a "bladder headache" starts at the top of the neck and goes up the head. The emotions with the Kidney and Bladder Meridian are fear and anxiety. The colors for the Kidney and Bladder Meridians are blue and black, the season is winter, and the time of day is three to seven PM.

The Liver Meridian is responsible for spreading the Qi through the body and for storing the Blood when we rest or sleep. It's related to the eyes, headaches, menstrual problems, vertigo, tendons, ligaments, the rib area, neck shoulders, tinnitus, spasms, strokes, depression, anger, and frustration. The Gallbladder Meridian works with the gallbladder (or the lack of the gallbladder). When it is out of balance, the skin, eyes, urine, and tongue can be tinted yellow. The emotion associated with this meridian is courage, and its time of night is eleven PM to three AM. The Liver and Gallbladder Meridians are associated with the spring season, and their color is green.

The Heart Meridian works with the blood vessels and moves the blood through them. Symptoms commonly seen with an imbalance here are insomnia, palpations, nightmares, skipping pulse, pain in the tongue, fever, and restlessness. The Small Intestine Meridian works with removing waste from the body. The related emotions are lack of joy or mania; the color is red, and its time of day is eleven AM to three PM.

The Heart Protection and Triple Warmer Meridians work with the Heart and Small Intestine Meridians. They are more difficult to explain because these meridians are not really organs, but rather they deal with the emotional aspects of the heart and the water system. Their time of night is from seven to eleven PM. They also have pulses, and their color is red.

The Spleen and Stomach Meridians come next, dealing with digestion in many ways. Their color is yellow, and their time of day is seven to eleven AM. Their emotion is sympathy or excessive worrying. Symptoms include weight gain or loss, phlegm, prolapsed organs, bleeding gums, bloating, weak or sore muscles, tumors, cysts, fibroids, and abnormal menstrual bleeding.

The last two meridians are called Ren and Du (or the conception vessel and governing vessel). These meridians connect with acupoints on many different levels. The meridians start on your feet and hands, travel up, down, and around your body. The conception vessel (Ren) and governing vessel (Du) run up the front and down the back, connecting around your mouth and anus. (Our treatments do not involve needling around the private parts, the mouth, or close to the eyes.)

Each meridian (except the Ren and Du Meridians) has its own flavor, color, sound, time of day, season, and emotion. There are strong and weak times of day for the meridians. As we listen to and examine you, we can decide which meridian requires treatment. Your skin color (whether red, green, yellow, white, or blue) and your emotional state help us to diagnose your health. People possess faint shades of color throughout their faces. For example, some people have dark circles under their eyes, and some people have red noses. We are trained to scan the whole face, along with the feet and hands, and note the coloring, which will correspond to different meridians. Shades of colors on parts of your face tell us volumes! Another factor we use in diagnosis is odor—because certain conditions have an odor. For example, bad breath tells us the Stomach Meridian is out of balance.

Every meridian has a pulse (except Ren and Du) with six pulses on each wrist, three deep and three on the surface. I mentally place each pulse in one of twenty-eight degrees or categories to help me identify the situation. I check them periodically to determine whether a patient is accepting the treatment.

What Is Balance?

If one word could describe acupuncture and Oriental medicine, it would be balance. Every bodily action or non-action (in and out) has one important function: to balance our bodies. This concept is called homeostasis.

The ancient Chinese knew that humans and the earth are all part of nature. What hurts one hurts the other; what heals one heals the other. The energy that flows through the body is similar to a flowing river. We suffer the same conditions that the earth does, for example, too much dampness, dryness, wind, cold, or heat.

When you have balance in your life, everything is better. You're happy and feel alive. You have the energy to do what you want and need to do. Your emotions also crave balance. Lifestyle changes, exercise, sleep, food, and water all help us to achieve this elusive balance. The ancient Chinese understood and wrote about this thousands of years ago. The human body and emotions haven't changed much since then, have they?

Maybe you recognize that your body and your emotions aren't quite in harmony. So you started reading this book and perhaps even made your first appointment for acupuncture. When you feel "out of balance," you should call your acupuncture physician.

The Chinese felt it was important to receive acupuncture treatment at least as often as the seasons changed (about every three months). Modern science tells us that most of our cells also renew themselves every three months. Coincidence? I don't think so!

What Is Qi?

Qi (pronounced chee) should be the easiest thing to write about because Qi is everything and everywhere. Qi is "energy," but also much more than energy. When you have enough Qi, you feel good. You are active, sleep well, think well, and everything seems to be going your way. When Qi is deficient, you wake up tired—if you were lucky enough to fall asleep. You don't want to eat, or you eat everything in sight, but mostly the wrong foods. For example, you might crave sugary or salty foods.

We can't see Qi, but we certainly see the results of Qi. Look at nature; you don't see the wind, but you do see the branches and leaves swaying. You can see water flowing down a stream. Did you ever wonder what moves the water? It is Qi.

Our bodies contain different types of Qi. Qi is in each cell and organ. We even inherit Qi, called Original Qi, from our parents, which is why it's a very good reason to obtain the best health possible before you conceive. Original Qi needs to last us through our lifetimes.

Another type of Qi, we receive GU Qi through our food, drink, and the air we breathe. The body takes Qi from the food and drink we ingest, then transforms, and transports it through the body to be used as Qi and Blood. When Qi flows in the right direction, we are fine, but if it reverses flow, we cough, hiccup, or vomit.

Qi moves freely throughout bodies except when we are not healthy, when it is stagnated. Symptoms of unhealthiness tell us there is a blockage and the Qi needs to be moved. The blockage can feel like a stabbing pain.

Each meridian has its own Qi. For example, when we breathe, the Lung Meridian grabs the air and sends it through the correct pathways where the Kidney Qi will pick it up. The Kidney Qi then separates the pure from the impure, and urine and carbon dioxide are formed. Urine is excreted through the kidneys and bladder, and carbon dioxide is expelled through exhaling.

As I've said, meridians run along our bodies like strands of Christmas tree lights. The energy's electrical aspect differs in places called acupoints. When needles are inserted in the acupoints, Qi can be moved, strengthened, or unblocked.

Qi is quite magnificent. As you receive treatments, you will learn to feel and identify Qi. You want to do all you can to increase your Qi. Eliminating your aches, pain, sensitivities, and allergies is a very good first step to bolstering Qi!

What Is Blood?

When we talk about Blood , we're not referring to the blood that you see when you accidentally cut yourself, but rather Blood as a form of Qi moving through your veins. Blood causes Qi to move with it. If you have pain that doesn't move from one area to another and is stabbing in nature, we say you have blood stagnation. If you feel weak or dizzy, have pale skin and lips and dry skin, and are losing your hair, you are most likely suffering from Blood deficiency. You can build your blood with acupuncture, food, herbs, and rest. Qi and Blood move and work together and need to be nourished to do this work.

What Are Yin and Yang?

You've probably heard of Yin and Yang and seen the Tai Ji symbol (the circle colored half black with a white dot and half white with a black dot). There is a little Yin in Yang and a little Yang in Yin as in ALL things. In the darkest of night comes a bit of light with the sun peeping over the horizon. Everyone has experienced "blinding light," a light so bright you can't see anything. Cold can be so cold that it feels hot and burns. You've heard the term *icy hot.*

There is a constant changing aspect to all things. These changes keep all things in balance. For example, women have many fluctuating female hormones with a little bit of male hormones. Men have many fluctuating male hormones with a little bit of female hormones.

Yin represents the female, cold, nighttime, moon, inside, interior, front, blood, bones, moistness, solid, softness, static, and deficient. Yang represents all of Yin's opposites: heat, daytime, sun, outside, exterior, back, Qi, skin, dryness, hollow, hardness, movement, and excess.

Chapter 3

Diagnosing Your Problem

Look, Listen, Smell, and Touch

I briefly mentioned in the preceding chapter how we diagnose problems and assist patients. When I explain to people that I want to know the color of their poop and its odor, I am serious. Each person has his/her unique bodily smell. Don't be embarrassed! I am never offended or disgusted because this information speaks volumes. I even observe how you walk, sit, move, and sound.

Pulse Diagnosis

The acupuncture physician will check your pulses, six on each wrist, which provides a better idea of your health. This technique goes back at least two thousand years and is based on the principle that Qi and Blood move through the body as one. Feeling the pulses is a learned art; a bad pulse is weak, very slow, slippery, and tight. A good pulse is even, strong, and smooth.

We place our hands on each wrist, gently press down a fraction of an inch, then let up, and feel the pulses on the surface. We can feel the blood coursing through the veins like anyone else taking your pulse would, but we also know that your Qi is the moving force of the blood.

We feel the strength, depth, width, force, rate, rhythm, size, and harmony of your pulses, and I look for excess and deficiency. If the pulse is pounding and trying to jump out of your skin, it's excess. If we can barely feel the pulse, it's deficient. More degrees of separations exist; in fact, each pulse can be present in twenty-seven different ways. In the summer, pulses tend to be more on the surface, and in the winter, they tend to be deeper. Children often have faster pulses than healthy adults.

I often provide patients with a chart outlining your pulses, which we can discuss at length. I also review your pulses during each visit, which is how I can tell if you're improving even if your symptoms fade away slowly. I can tell if you are tired or had too much caffeine or a cigarette recently. Although I have taken postgraduate classes and read more than ten books on the subject (one of which has over 700 pages), I would never say I am an expert on pulse diagnosis.

Pulse diagnosis is a strange concept to anyone in the Western world, especially medical personnel who have taken pulses on patients in a hospital or doctor's office. I was one of those people. However, after checking pulses on thirty patients one morning, I KNEW there were twelve pulses! The hard part is interpreting them.

One teacher told me that the Chinese practitioners feel you can't really know how to interpret a pulse until you have done it for twenty-seven years! Hopefully, in another thirteen years, I will be "really" good at it!

I check pulses two to three times during a treatment. When patients leave, their pulses are much better than when they came in. For patients who come in at least every three months, I can feel an improvement that doesn't diminish much unless they "come down with something" or have a major health challenge.

On a pregnant woman, practitioners can feel a quality that resembles two pulses inside. We call it slippery—not the same slippery as someone with a cold though. It feels like running your fingers over a dish of pearls.

Tongue Diagnosis

Tongue diagnosis dates back to the Shang Dynasty (1600 BC to 1000 BC). Many books focus on tongue diagnosing, and those who study acupuncture and Oriental medicine spend a great deal of time in school learning about tongues.

The appearance of your tongue gives a good indication of your organs' health. Your tongue can change in appearance daily. A tongue can have white gooey stuff on it, or it can be any shade from yellow to brown. It can have scalloped edges, a raw tip, be swollen, thin, dry, or have moist quivers or any combination of the above. If the tongue is short, acupuncture physicians know there is a Cold condition in the body. If it is too long, there is heat. Cracks on your tongue can indicate a deficiency of the B complex or zinc.

The color of your tongue tells us if you're suffering from anemia; if it's pale or dark purplish red, you may lack enough of the vitamin B complex. A purple tongue also hints of stagnation. A pale tongue tells acupuncture physicians of a Cold condition. A scalloped tongue can mean a zinc deficiency and most certainly a Spleen Qi deficiency. A shiny tongue can indicate a lack of B12. Thick white fur shows an acupuncture physician that there is too much phlegm and the stomach is not operating correctly and can also be a sign of Candida. Dark yellow fur indicates a heat and phlegm condition with poor stomach action. A thick tongue illustrates that the adrenal glands are not properly functioning and need support. A bright red tongue with no fur tells us there is "stomach heat." A dry tongue indicates depleted fluids, and a moist one shows there is poor fluid transportation. Tongues that quiver tell us that you don't have enough Qi to hold your tongue still. Additionally some tongues look raw; and some are dark red or pale.

The tongue is a map to the body. The heart is on the tip, and the kidney, bladder, and large and small intestines are in the back; the lungs are located behind the heart before the spleen and stomach, and on the sides are the liver and gallbladder. The stomach and spleen are behind the heart in the middle. Acupuncture Physicians can decipher much helpful information from your tongue.

Chapter 4

Office Visits— Treatment Begins

Oriental medicine and acupuncture have an individualistic and complex approach to diagnosis and treatment. You will be examined and treated as a whole body, not just a gallbladder or back pain. Before you meet with your acupuncture physician, you will be asked to complete an extensive health questionnaire. Feel free to bring lists of medicines, vitamins, herbs, surgeries, or test results from other physicians you have seen.

The acupuncture physician will review your questionnaire before he/she meets with you. As she walks into the room, she will observe your skin color. Is your skin red, pale, tinged with yellow, dark around your eyes, or gray around your mouth?

Next the acupuncture physician will listen. This is your time to discuss everything that concerns you. You are not complaining but explaining. We want to hear your story in your own words. As you talk, we will listen to the sound and strength of your voice and your breathing. We will notice how you sit, if you rub sore areas as you talk, how you get up, and how you move around.

Next you will be shown to a treatment room that is a very comfortable temperature. The room will have a padded table and soft music. Here you will remove your shoes and socks and lie down on your back. You will rest for a few minutes, hopefully relaxing a little.

Your acupuncture physician will check your pulse and look at your tongue. After examining you, the acupuncture physician will begin your treatment. She will wipe off twelve or so spots (acupoints) with alcohol and then insert needles. Usually the needles are inserted only a fraction of an inch. The needles are typically placed on your hands, arms, legs, and feet. However, a needle may be placed between your eyebrows for relaxation or a few may be positioned in your ear.

The needles are solid, not hollow like hypodermic needles. They are flexible and are as skinny as a strand of hair. They may have a plastic, colored handle that indicates the needle's size. When the needles are inserted, you may feel a little sting, similar to a mosquito bite. Rarely does the insertion of the needle cause pain, but be sure to let someone know if there is pain after the needles are in your skin.

The acupuncture physician will check your pulses again and leave the room, which will be peaceful and dimly lit. If you wish, you may be covered with a special blanket that will not touch the needles. Always let the staff know what you need to be comfortable. You will usually remain in the room during the treatment for twenty to thirty minutes. Your pulses determine how long your treatment will be. When the acupuncture physician decides your treatment is finished, she will remove the needles by giving them a slight pull or twist. The removal may occur so quickly that you don't see it. This removal technique is called manipulation, and it pulls the Qi up (see the section on needles). Your Acupuncture Physician will decide how many visits will be needed to correct your problem. This is based on the information gathered from your first visit.

In Our Clinic

At this point of your visit in our clinic you and I decide if you are a candidate for the AcuSET treatments. If you are, I will explain the computerized testing and schedule an appointment for the next available testing day, usually within a week.

If your pain is related to an injury or chronic condition, we will proceed with the treatments unless secondary symptoms that are sensitivity/allergy related are present, in which case we may combine treatments. If you are in a very weakened state, we may use acupuncture for a few weeks to strengthen you and then do the AcuSET treatments. I strengthen patients with acupuncture before AcuSET treatments about 10 percent of the time.

If we have determined you need to be treated with the AcuSET procedure, then you will also be tested on this visit. At the end of this visit, we will discuss the test results and all information I have gathered during the first two visits. You will also receive an acupuncture treatment (see chapter 5).

Your second visit will focus on testing to determine if and identify what sensitivities are affecting you. As we proceed with the electrodermal computerized screening test (EDS or Food and Environmental Sensitivity Assessment (FESA)), you may ask questions, although sitting back and relaxing is beneficial as well. We can stop and take a break if you need to, and I often encourage patients to drink water during a testing break.

When the test is completed—usually after about a half hour—you will be directed to a treatment room. When I join you, I will explain your test findings and the approximate number of visits needed to correct the sensitivities. Together we will review the symptoms that brought you to our clinic. The acupuncture treatment will be similar to the one you received on the first visit, but this time treatment vials will be introduced. The vials are in a sealed, glass jar, which will be placed near you. You don't have to hold the vials, but rather just relax and enjoy your acupuncture treatment!

Nutritional Assessment

On the first or second visit, I will explain the online health questionnaire that will be emailed to you. After the initial consultation and/or treatment, some patients realize they suffer from additional issues. This questionnaire helps us to put your whole picture together, including your current nutritional status. Remember you are not complaining but explaining to us what is happening in your life. If you don't have access to email or choose not to use the computer, you can also take the forms home with you.

We always like to know what supplements you take, and we may change your dosage, add additional supplements, or discourage you from taking other supplements depending upon the best course of treatment for you. I find people tend to take more supplements than they need.

Computerized Meridian Assessments

Albert Einstein proved that everything is energy and energy is everything. Our brains and nervous systems measure energy on a constant basis. Different energy patterns distinguish objects from each other. Colors, smells, foods, people, animals, plants, and anything we can touch, see, feel, or smell has energy. An x-ray shows a broken bone by measuring energy. An EKG measures the heartbeat, while EEG measures brainwaves. We do not see the actual wave in our brain but a computerized readout of the energy. If something is blocking the energy, it is called an impedance.

Thousands of points on the body have been scientifically documented to correspond to different organs or systems in the body. These points have a lowered electrical resistance. In the 1990s, MRI studies showed that when a certain acupuncture point was touched, the part of the brain that registers vision would react. That point, Liver 3, is in fact used by acupuncturists to treat eye problems.

Accordingly, computerized meridian assessment is used in our clinic. For the test, you sit in a comfortable chair placing your hand on a curved "plate." You will feel nothing as the computer is reading the lower electrical resistance and translating the information for the physician. When your hand is on the plate a small amount of battery power travels through that point and the impedance (or resistance) of that energy tells us if there is a weakness or excess, based on a scale of 0-100. The information gathered from your body is analyzed. Your acupuncturist then has more complete data regarding your health. This test is inexpensive and is available at your request or my determination. As with all other equipment in our clinic, it is FDA registered.

Electrodermal Computerized Testing

It's well established that the heart produces electrical energy that is reflected through other tissue to the skin of the chest where it can be measured through an EKG. Measuring this energy is a useful way to determine some normal or abnormal functions of the heart and is performed during a comprehensive medical examination. In a similar fashion, the electrical energy of the brain is reflected through the relatively dense bone of the head to the skin of the skull where it can also be measured through an EEG. Similar measurements are conducted through Electromyography and Brain Stem Audiometry tests.

It should not be surprising then that other organs can reflect their energy components to the skin at various locations. However, the energy that travels through connective tissue under the skin from one conventional acupuncture point to another is a bit harder to "pin" down, if you'll excuse the pun.

Experiments in which a classical acupuncture point is injected with a radioactive substance and then followed have established that the radioactive substance can be quickly traced from that acupuncture point, flowing in one direction only, to the next point in the classical meridian pathway, which was established some three thousand years earlier. Amazingly, the ancient Chinese identified these points accurately and functionally connected specific points with specific organ systems, and they did so long before our current concepts of blood circulation, nerve pathways, and other anatomical knowledge and without the use of x-ray, MRI, or other modern investigative tools.

As you may have experienced, an electrical charge introduced into a human body (for example, touching an electrified fence, a car battery cable, or other AC electrical source) can cause a significant shock. Anyone else touching that person at that time may also feel the shock. A few years ago, I witnessed an interesting demonstration in which two people held on to the metal contact points in the paws of a toy teddy bear that talked when the paws were touched together. Nearly a hundred other people joined them to hold each other's hands in a large circle. When the circle was complete, the teddy bear spoke. When someone at the far end of the circle let go of his neighbor's hand, the speaking stopped. When they again held hands, the talking teddy bear resumed speaking. All those people formed an electrical circuit powered by a tiny battery in the teddy bear.

When a patient is tested by the computerized electrodermal screening for the AcuSET protocol equipment, he or she holds a moistened brass rod in one hand while the technician touches an acupuncture point with a probe connected to the machine. This action creates a circuit with a very small, unfelt current running through the patient. The amount of resistance experienced at that point or the amount of current flowing (conductance) can be measured. The patient feels nothing more than a little pressure. The test can be stopped at any time if it's uncomfortable, but this rarely happens.

Abnormal readings inform the acupuncture physician about that acupoint and its associated organ system. Further, a substance, even something in a glass jar that is introduced into this electrical circuit may change the acupoint's reading in a helpful or harmful way. Imagine the benefit of knowing if an anesthetic may harm a patient about to undergo surgery, if an implant or dental material may react badly if used by a particular patient, or if a patient who has a reaction to a needed drug could determine if another medication may be more compatible.

In addition to measuring the resistance in a point, simply touching a particular point on a given meridian can make a previously strong muscle temporarily weak. This would indicate a problem in the meridian's energy component and possibly in its corresponding organ system. If touching a point while bringing a possible allergenic substance into close proximity causes the previously strong muscle to become weak, then this would indicate that the body does not do as well when close to that substance.

Many clinicians use this muscle-testing procedure to determine compatibility to a given substance. Effective muscle testing, or applied kinesiology, requires good technique and lots of experience. I choose to use the computerized electrodermal screening equipment from two of the leading manufacturers of bioelectrical impedance measurement devices. Over three thousand medical doctors, chiropractors, physicians, acupuncture physicians, and other health care practitioners use the equipment, which are registered with the U.S. Food & Drug Administration. I find the devices' color-coded reports to be reliable and easily understood by my patients. After treating thousands of patients, I find the equipment are just as reliable as they were eleven years ago, although I always search for the best, most up-to-date equipment for my patients' care.

When patients come to us, they typically want to know four things:
1. Can acupuncture help me?
2. What's wrong with me?
3. How many visits will I need?
4. What will this cost?

After gathering the needed facts, I will be able to diagnose your condition and can estimate the cost and number of visits. If I accept you as a patient, I am very sure acupuncture will help you—at the least acupuncture will improve the quality of your life.

Missed Appointments

If you can't keep your appointment, we need to know as soon as possible. We don't charge for missed appointments; I count on your consideration and respect for others. Please don't change your appointment with us because "something" came up, such as a visiting friend or relative or another changed appointment. Your visit entails an important procedure, which you need to commit to for your overall well-being. You can bring your friends and/or relatives with you, and we will be happy to explain acupuncture to them.

You may always check with me before you leave regarding your next appointment. I keep a copy of your calendar in your file. I will also know if you skip appointments. Missing appointments can slow your progress. Each treatment builds on the previous ones. If you miss three appointments, you and I will discuss your case, and you may be RELEASED FROM CARE. I can't help you if you don't want to help yourself. These techniques work, but you need to be here to receive them.

Chapter 5

Instruments Used for Treatments

Needles

Early in acupuncture's history, acupuncturists used bone, bronze (1760 BC), tin, copper, silver, or gold needles. Although modern acupuncturists use stainless steel needles, their needling techniques are based on information written around 600 AD.

Acupuncture physicians insert needles into the skin at specific acupoint areas. The acupuncturist will gently manipulate the small needles a few times during your session and remove them in a certain way. The procedure may look very simple, but in fact, much technique occurs in the insertion and removal of the needles. When we insert the needle, we very gently rotate the needle in a counterclockwise or clockwise movement. We may push it down or pull it up a fraction of an inch. The needle's manipulation activates the Qi. The acupuncture physician feels a "tug" (called Deqi) on the needle, which is somewhat like a fish nibbling on a fishing line. The Deqi tells us that we have arrived at our objective.

You might feel a sensation or slight pressure. The movement of Qi throughout your body takes approximately fifteen to twenty minutes, but is based on your breathing. The average treatment is twenty minutes. Some conditions require a tonification treatment, which is shorter than a sedation treatment, which can take up to forty-five minutes.

At the acupuncture school I attended, we took classes in theory and point location before we inserted even one needle. Five months after we started classes, we took a test developed by the Centers for Disease Control. We could not perform needling until we successfully passed this test. Several years later, I have inserted over 500,000 needles.

The needles are classified as filiform, meaning they are solid. They have a very sharp point, are flexible, and come in different lengths and gauges. We use needles from .5 to 1.5 inches long and gauges of 27 to 31 in our practice (about the width of a hair). We use approximately twelve needles on each visit, but that varies with your condition.

Needling doesn't occur the way you see it portrayed in movies. The needles are inserted just under the skin after the area is cleaned off with alcohol. We always wash our hands and use an antiseptic cleaner right before we touch you.

There may be a slight prickly feeling on insertion, but it does not last. If at any time you are uncomfortable, please let us know. The acupuncture treatment is normally a very pleasant experience, and most people fall asleep.

Very rarely, you may notice a small bruise after the treatment. This symptom could indicate a problem with your body. Some prescription medicines cause a person to bruise easily, which is one reason we ask for a list of the medicines you take. A bruise can indicate other health conditions, but most of the time, it's just a bruise. However, please bring it to our attention on your next visit. You can put an ice cube on it when you get home.

Upon completion of your treatment, the needles are placed in a biohazard waste container that any doctor's office contains. We pay a biohazard waste control company to dispose of the needles. We are also inspected by the state on a yearly basis for safety and sanitary precautions and always pass inspection 100 percent.

Cupping and Gua Sha

Cupping helps regulate the flow of Qi and Blood. It draws out Wind, Cold, Heat, and Dampness in the body. Cupping is good for pains, problems with the digestive, circulatory and respiratory systems, weakness in muscles, high blood pressure, common colds, and chest congestion. It can also be used on joints to increase the activity of synovial fluid and blood.

Written records of cupping date back to 2500 BC. The procedure has been used all over the world, and some of my patients even remember their Italian moms doing it to them as children. The cups are about the size of juice glasses. We clean the skin off with alcohol and place the cup over it. We squeeze the attached suction device until it feels tight around the area but not uncomfortable. We will apply three or four cups at a time. After a few minutes, we gently rock the cup, and it comes off. Sometimes a reddish ring or spot will linger, which is perfectly normal. As the patient, you'll only feel a gentle pulling on your skin. Cupping is not unpleasant but rather relaxing, and it takes just a few minutes.

A very low-pressure pull occurs during the procedure, caused by the response of the blood vessels within the muscles to the stimulation of the blood vessels just below the skin. This movement in the muscles allows the flow of blood and feels like a gentle pulling.

Some experts believed that early physicians invented cupping as a procedure to suck poison from wounds. Some of the first cups were gourds, and eventually, glass cups were introduced. Nineteenth-century doctors in Europe and the United States used cupping for a variety of illnesses. The procedure still enjoys popularity in Asia. However, cupping isn't for everyone; for example, I wouldn't use the procedure on people with very fine or dry skin.

After the treatment, the skin can be pink or red for a while because of the rise in skin temperature and the increase of blood flow. Physicians can perform cupping safely over lung areas and along the back to aid internal organs. I once treated an exotic dancer who would only let us apply the cups to areas of her body that she knew would be covered. She said the cupping helped pain in her legs and she asked for it at least once a month.

In my second month of acupuncture school, our teacher explained a popular technique called Gua Sha. To understand how it works, we must refer back to the chapter that discussed Blood. Blood is a form of Qi produced by the spleen, transported by the lungs, and transformed by the heart. Blood nourishes and moistens the body and flows with Qi throughout the body. And Blood also may become stuck and cause pain—Blood stagnation.

A trained practitioner performs Gua Sha by gently running a ceramic soupspoon along your back, neck, and arms after applying a liniment for gliding ease. We use a short stroke with the spoon similar to petting a cat. The Sha appears along the areas we rub and indicates Blood stagnation. The Sha can be light to dark red and will fade in a day or so. Patients report immediate relief and looseness in the area.

Your acupuncture physician can show you how to perform Gua Sha at home. This technique is not formally taught in Chinese schools, but rather it is something a Chinese mother would do if her child came down with a cold or had a stiff neck. Experiencing Gua Sha is very pleasant, but the results may look like a hickey on your body. In fact, in the 1970s, the marks on Asian children in California who attended school after receiving Gua Sha would often cause their teachers to report child abuse.

I was so amazed by this technique that I spent forty dollars for a thin book on Gua Sha and excitedly told my Chinese teacher, who was mystified by my reaction. She said my grandmother could have told me all I needed to know about Gua Sha. She was surprised when I told her that Americans didn't know anything about Gua Sha.

Moxibustion

Every day a patient, after seeing moxibustion in a movie or talk show, asks me about burning an herb on the end of a needle. Popular in China, moxibustion is a modality that treats and prevents disease by introducing heat to the acupoints. The practitioner takes a rolled-up portion of herbs and lights it on top of a needle. The resulting heat helps the herbal properties to be drawn into the body. A famous doctor, Ge Hong, wrote a book sometime during the Jin Dynasty (AD 317-420) describing ninety-nine different conditions that use moxibustion.

Artemisia vulgaris, the most commonly used herb, belongs to the chrysanthemum family. When it is burned, the heat penetrates the body through the acupoints and meridians. It then activates the Qi and Blood circulation, breaks up stagnation and swelling, and eliminates cold and dampness.

In the United States, we mostly use a cigar-shaped roll of compressed artemisia vulgaris. It is lit and held a few inches from the skin and can be placed over a needle. The herb has contraindications such as pregnancy, the thin skin of elderly people, and high fevers. Some practitioners including myself prefer to use a special lamp with a spray version of the herb. Artemisia vulgaris has a very strong odor, and people with allergies and sensitivities can't handle the smell. We also use a moxa warmer with a salve. It's very safe and extremely effective, and there is no odor.

Acupuncture physicians follow a carefully planned treatment protocol derived from years of research and knowledge of biochemistry and acupuncture. You will receive a copy of your records, which will help you become more involved in the treatment process. Reading this book will also facilitate your understanding of what is happening and why. Please feel free to ask questions anytime. It may help to write down your questions and bring them with you.

Safety and Possible Adverse Reactions

People with health problems tend to be "toxic." A poor diet, overconsumption of alcohol, lack of exercise, and poor bowel habits are all negatives. Acupuncture brings the body back to health.

If you experience mild or uncomfortable symptoms during your treatments, toxicity can be an explanation. Symptoms such as mild nausea, tiredness, muscle aches, headaches, food cravings, itchiness, and anxiety are rare but can occur. We can help with a mild homeopathic detoxification program. This inexpensive program can easily be incorporated with your treatments. The detoxification can take place in a few different ways, such as a fruit and vegetable diet with some gentle herbal medicines or a homeopathic program with medicine that you would drink for a few days. Neither method is unpleasant or dangerous and people feel much better, faster.

To ease your mind further, a recently released study regarding the safety of acupuncture needles found that there have only been fifty reports of infections from needling in the last forty years. I am extremely careful and practice guidelines set by the CDC (Centers for Disease Control) as do all acupuncture physicians in the United States.

Chapter 6

What Does Acupuncture Treat?

The World Health Organization is the authority concerning health-related matters across the world. Since 1992, the WHO has published a list of (what is now) sixty-eight symptoms, conditions, diseases, pathologies, and traumas that have been definitively and effectively treated by acupuncture. Below I have listed many of the conditions that acupuncture can improve or eliminate.

Allergies and Food Sensitivities

Allergies and food sensitivities can manifest in many different ways, but always entail a reaction to a food eaten, smelled, or touched. People with food sensitivities feel like they are classic hypochondriacs. Some individuals react negatively if they are within inches of touching a particular item. Some complain of feeling bloated or of puffiness around the eyes and nose. These reactions could be caused by the body's confused and overactive immune system surrounding the cells with a watery substance to flush away the invaders (normally harmless items). As a result, cells become waterlogged and tissues (typically hands, ankles, and feet) swell. Another common reaction is sneezing and a runny nose. Some of my patients have had a constantly runny nose when they eat. Others experience rapid heartbeats or drowsiness. Unfortunately, it's not unusual to experience symptoms and not link them to sensitivities.

What causes allergies and food sensitivities? Well, people eat more wheat, corn, milk, and eggs than ever before. If we look at the typical diet, we see an increase in fast foods, restaurant foods, and commercially prepared foods. These foods usually contain extra fat, fillers, additives, and chemicals. Studies prove that these food items cause most of the reactions and symptoms.

How are we going to digest and assimilate genetically altered food? Not too well, I'm sure. When human bodies "showed up" millions of years ago, they expected to eat naturally occurring foods. We ate fruit, vegetables, nuts, fish and wild-game meats. Milk and wheat were not introduced into the human diet until ten thousand years ago. Sugar wasn't eaten much until the 1900s.

We have evolved and adapted, but not quickly enough to handle the food changes in the last thirty years. When I started studying nutrition in the seventies, it was estimated we each ate fifty pounds of sugar a year; today, the number is 155 pounds per year—quite an increase!

We have five immunoglobulins in our blood serum. They are similar but different. They protect us from invaders such as viruses, bacteria, and allergic reactions. When your body thinks something strange has invaded it, it goes into attack mode and eventually creates antibodies against the invaders, which can be bacteria, viruses, a food, or a chemical; the antibodies are protein molecules or immunoglobulins.

Our bodies start to protect us at birth. Food allergy symptoms generally don't occur immediately (except in the case of anaphylactic reactions) due to the release of the IgE to the cells. Reactions can take up to three days to appear because the IgG antibodies continue circulating throughout the body. IgE and IgG are the different types of protein molecules that register allergic responses.

Food cravings also are a common sensitivity symptom. People complain of being "addicted" to certain foods. One patient ate a dozen eggs a day. Guess what? That was her top sensitivity. Another patient ate handfuls of salt every day; her leading sensitivity was salt. When you eat the offending food, your body releases brain chemicals that cause a good feeling.

When you quit eating the food, you may experience uncomfortable or strong reactions, so your brain tells you to eat it again. For example, it is not unusual for someone to come in to our clinic complaining of migraines that occur every week. I had a male patient who suffered like this daily. He vomited nightly for hours, which would stop the headaches until the next morning. Another patient suffered like this, alternating between vomiting and migraine headaches, for more than twenty years.

I believe we develop allergies and sensitivities because we don't have a correctly working digestive system with the right enzymes to process our food. Whole natural foods contain the proper enzymes to promote digestion but processing kills the enzymes. For example, after age forty, we produce less hydrochloric acid. A symptom of this is heartburn or an acidy taste in the mouth. People think they have too much acid when this happens, but the opposite is true.

They will then take an antacid, their problems become worse, and eventually they will be placed on prescription medicines.

Other digestive factors include eating too much at once, eating under stress, general stress, not chewing correctly, drinking too many liquids with meals, drinking cold or iced liquids, and eating too many cold or raw foods. From the perspective of Oriental medicine, studying during meals pulls the Spleen Qi away from its job of transporting nutrients; mealtime needs to be a calm and relaxing time to enjoy your food without cell phones, work, or unpleasant conversation.

Some reports state that sixty percent of adults suffer from food sensitivities. Additionally, some experts say food sensitivities have increased over 35 percent in the last twenty years. Food allergies are less common and are identified by a blood test or a scratch test on the skin. You do not need these tests to tell you that you reacted in a negative way to something you ate recently or used in preparing a meal.

Patients almost always visit their physicians for the symptoms above, and their physicians diagnose them and prescribe the proper medication. However, Oriental medicine approaches and explains some of these symptoms differently, and as an acupuncture physician, I use AcuSET to treat food sensitivities instead of medications.

When one female patient came to our office with a myriad of physical ailments, I asked her, "Is anything working right in your body?" She recently sent this letter:

> *Dear Rusty, Again I want to thank you for literally saving my life. My allergic reactions and my autoimmune system were destroying my body. Thank God, I found your advertisement in*

a Natural Awakening *magazine and made an appointment for a consultation and acupuncture treatment. Your AcuSET has worked wonders/miracles in my body and in my life overall. I have ZERO allergic reactions. My eyes have improved tremendously. My prescription for glasses is extremely less than before. My eye doctor said he has seen this kind of improvement before due to acupuncture treatments in patients. My lab reports are considerably better than before. My blood sugar/glucose labs improved (previously 113 to 99); my blood sugar/insulin levels improved (previous 167 to presently 44). Some other changes have also taken place. Each time I get acupuncture, improvements are shown. —BJH*

We have many more of these letters in our files from people that could not eat Thanksgiving dinner for fear of severe reactions that may send them to the ER. One patient could only eat the same six things for months. She was exhausted and lost quite a bit of weight. She could not work or get out of bed most days. The emotional toll was horrible. Unfortunately, all of her trouble started after a reaction to an antibiotic.

However, acupuncture routinely causes positive improvements for people suffering from food sensitivities, which is why this treatment has lasted thousands of years. With proven results throughout the centuries, why aren't millions of people trying acupuncture daily?

Anxiety

Anxiety causes panic attacks, shakiness, palpitations, racing heart, hyperventilation, dizziness, headaches, diarrhea, vomiting, unexplained fears, feelings of dread, and insomnia. Sufferers can't calm down and feel like they lack control over their lives. In Oriental medicine, this pattern of symptoms is usually connected to the Heart, Liver, and Kidney Meridians.

Anxiety also involves a deficiency of Qi, Blood, Yin, and Yang. The most common causes of anxiety are sensitivities to food colorings, additives, sugar, alcohol, and the vitamin B complex. After sensitivities are eliminated through acupuncture treatment, people who complain of anxiety are calmer and sleep better. We also provide instruction to patients on breathing techniques, exercise, and proper diet to help improve their lifestyles. We also use homeopathic and herbal medicines for anxiety. We commonly treat anxiety with successful results.

Arthritis

The top two reasons people seek help from acupuncture is for arthritis and allergies. The third reason is infertility and the fourth is stress. I was surprised to learn that food sensitivities could cause pain and inflammation. In Oriental medicine, joints are the place where Qi and Blood gather. When Heat, Cold, Dampness, and Wind attack, they cause a painful obstruction. Called Bi Syndromes, two types of this condition exist: Cold Bi Syndrome and Hot Bi Syndrome. The patient usually knows if their joint pain feels hot or cold. Alternatively, if heat feels good on the joint, it is the cold type. In Western medicine, the cold type of arthritis is classified as wear and tear on joints and degeneration of articular cartilages such as knee, hip, ankle, wrist, and finger joints. As time goes by, there can be pain, stiffness, and inflammation.

My husband had been a runner for thirty-five years without any problems. Eleven years ago, he showed me his feet; they were almost purple and felt very hot. He complained of pain, something he never did! He suspected allergies to bananas and wheat were causing these symptoms. I thought he was crazy, but he made an appointment for allergy tests. The tests came back with twenty-five of the fifty items showing positive for moderately severe allergies.

I was still unsure about the connection between arthritis pain and food allergies, but I agreed not to feed him those twenty-five items—and they were good foods, not junk foods! After a couple of weeks, he felt a little better but not enough to make either of us happy. I started buying bananas again; I figured I didn't have arthritis pain so I could eat them, but his symptoms got worse! About this time, I learned about NAET, and both of us decided to try it.

We also continued to treat my husband for the foods on his list, and he gradually got better. Three months later, we tested him using the computerized electrodermal screening equipment. The items that we had treated him for tested at zero, meaning no reaction to them; the items for which we had not treated him were still reactive. In the next two weeks, we treated him for everything that showed up in previous blood tests and the items we identified from the electrodermal screenings. Eleven years later, and he hasn't had that pain since.

Rheumatoid Arthritis

One of my patients could not drive, dress herself, shop, clean her house, or cook due to rheumatoid arthritis (RA). She spent most of the day sitting in a chair. All day long, her pain level would be ten—unbearable—on a scale of one to ten. She took seven medications and suffered from depression. We had difficulty getting her up on the table, but she insisted on lying down for the treatments.

She would curl up in the fetal position as she could not lie straight. I treated her with acupuncture for two weeks. She noticed a little pain relief but was still in a very bad state.

I described to her what I had done for other RA patients. She said she had nothing to lose, so we tested her for food sensitivities. She had quite a number of food sensitivities, and her reaction numbers were quite high. We proceeded to see each other two times a week for the next three weeks. The weekend after Thanksgiving, she called me at home and told me she had done dishes for the first time in twenty-five years. "I'll see you on Monday," she said, "and I might drive myself." When I saw her, her fingers weren't as curled as they had been and she was on less pain medicine, but more importantly, she felt like a person again.

Another woman who had been diagnosed with rheumatoid arthritis a few years earlier approached me after one of my lectures. She was in severe daily pain. She worked and cared for her family and tried to keep a workout schedule. She was on a lot of medication and was not happy with their side effects. I explained that my practice had had success with rheumatoid arthritis, but that we would need to examine and test her before determining if we could help. My staff rearranged my morning appointments so she could come in the next morning (it usually takes a about a week to get an appointment for testing). We found multiple sensitivities and started treatment that day. She started receiving pain relief after a couple of weeks. I find that most people start to see results in two weeks. At the end of six weeks, she was very pleased.

One remarkable symptom about this woman was the intense heat coming from her fingers. I could actually feel it six inches from her hand. As time went on, the heat and the pain both decreased.

After the initial schedule of treatments, we both agreed that she needed to continue to visit twice a month. During this time, she had a previously scheduled appointment with her physician. She was able to show him greater range of motion and reduced swelling. She told him she was for the most part pain-free and that the heat in her hands was gone. He said he was glad the medicines worked; she told him she had quit taking them (I didn't know this) months earlier and was using acupuncture. He was not pleased and told her she would come crawling back for her pain medications very soon.

She hasn't yet, and it has been four years now. She comes for treatment every other month for a "tune-up," and the first thing I check is the heat in her hands. It has never come back!

This spring a seventy-eight-year-old woman came in using a walker and bent over in pain, although she was on heavy medications. She could only stand for a few minutes and had trouble sitting. She also has rheumatoid arthritis and lupus, had a stroke twenty years previous, and was partially paralyzed on the right side. But her severe pain only began about two years before. We treated her with acupuncture and scheduled a return visit in one week. I called her the next day. She told me that she was able to stand up and had very little pain. I was skeptical! The next day a friend of hers came in and told me the same thing except now this patient was walking with a cane. Acupuncture doesn't always prompt results like hers, but it is worth a try. Some pain relief would be a blessing. I checked on her a couple of months later; she was in some pain that had returned just a few days before and wanted to come in every month for treatment.

There are different types of arthritis: rheumatoid, lupus, osteoarthritis, and ankylosing spondylitis (arthritis of the spine).

I have treated patients with all three types in various degrees of pain and inflammation with good to excellent results. Most of my patients over sixty think or know they have arthritis, which is treated quite well with acupuncture.

Asthma

In Oriental medicine, we use the term *asthmatic breathing* to describe a patient who has trouble breathing with some wheezing. This term is different from the medical diagnosis of asthma. Clinical definitions of asthma indicate inflammation of the airways with coughing, chest tightness, wheezing, and trouble inhaling and exhaling.

The Lung Meridian governs the function of breathing and protecting the skin. The Lung Meridian is easily affected by wind and cold, heat and dryness. "Asthmatic" patients endure many more symptoms with greater severity than others do with the flu or a cold. They cannot take in a breath or exhale. Unless you have experienced this disorder, you cannot imagine the panic that patients suffering from asthmatic breathing feel.

I have successfully treated many asthmatic cases. I never tell these patients to stop taking their medicines or inhalers. In fact, my first asthmatic patient finally threw hers away as it had expired five years ago. I checked with her last week, and she has not had any lung issues in nine years.

Studies show that asthmatics can be helped by including magnesium and fish oils in their diets. Sometimes eliminating gluten or diary can help. Acupuncture and chiropractic treatment does work to relieve the symptoms and sometimes the entire problem as seen below.

One very chilly day in January two years ago, I walked into a treatment room to see my next patient. I instantly realized I did not know this patient and that she was having trouble breathing. I took her pulse and said that I needed to call 911. She said she wouldn't go if I did call an ambulance because they couldn't do much more for her. She had driven more than forty-five minutes by herself to my office. I quickly inserted the needles for breathing problems and sat down next to her to monitor her breathing, knowing I'd be calling 911 in a few minutes. In about fifteen minutes, she started to breathe more normally. She told me that she was feeling less tightness in her chest and would be fine. We were able to do a full new-patient evaluation. Here is her story:

> *I had suffered from asthma and allergies for over sixty-five years. I had tried all the treatments that any allergist could offer. One day in January 2005, I woke up and could not breathe. I realized I had a few minutes to reach my inhaler and get some air to my lungs. Finally, I could breathe but was faced with the problem of getting emergency help.*
>
> *I was alone as my husband was out of town. Miracles happen. My phone rang, and it was Debra Gaffney's office. I had been waiting for an appointment. I told them I could not come in as I was having a major asthma attack. The voice on the other end of the phone said, "We can take care of that." Within the hour, I was there, and Debra proceeded very cautiously to do acupuncture on me. I was so ill I didn't mind that I had never had acupuncture before.*
>
> *About fifteen minutes later, I felt such relief. I had the feeling that a huge elephant had gotten off my chest finally!*

I could breathe! I had never had such relief that quickly before. Through testing, I learned I was sensitive to some of the stuff I was taking to help my asthma.

I still see Debra sometimes as a new problem will come up, and my lungs are still slightly weakened. I can now eat tomatoes and strawberries, go to homes that have dogs, cats, or birds, walk every day, breathe the air, and do almost anything I could never do most of my life. I am a new person inside. I am no longer mentally confused. I think clearer; I feel healthier. I have no reflux problems, allergies, or asthma.

**Update: This patient is doing quite well.
I see her a few times a year for a tune-up.**

In my first month of practice, a local doctor referred one of his asthmatic patients to me. This pleasant lady was a retired massage therapist and "wanted to do things in a more natural way." We conducted the Meridian Stress Assessment and the Food and Environmental Sensitivity Assessment. Her Lung and Kidney Meridians were weakened. The Spleen and Liver Meridians were in an excess state. The patient also complained of lots of phlegm, anxiety attacks, diarrhea, and stomach problems. I treated her for the next six months with remarkable results. Her extraordinary testimonial is on our website.

Strange things happened to some people after the hurricanes in Florida in 2004. They developed allergies and asthma for the first time. The only explanation I had was the presence of trees, weeds, flowers, and plants that were chewed up and distributed in other parts of the state. A few months after the hurricanes, I noticed a weed I had not seen before. I checked the "weed" book and found the plant came from a different part of the state. I developed a cough that was so severe I couldn't sleep. I carried this weed to our agriculture center for some advice. By the time the master gardener came out to see me, I couldn't talk at all! I went home, held that weed, and gave myself a treatment. The next day I was fine.

A woman who suffered greatly after the hurricanes and was on medicine for her whole life was referred to me by one of her relatives. Her CT scan showed problems in her lungs. She suffered with coughs, sinus pressure, chest tightness, breathing problems, and headaches. Ten days after her treatment started, she went off her medicines. Again, I do not encourage this and even caution against it. She finished her course of treatment, and one year later is fine. Another CT scan showed great improvement.

Six years ago, a man from Wisconsin showed up on our doorstep for treatment of allergies and asthma. His dad had heard a woman at the post office telling another woman about our treatments. He was only going to be here a week or so. He kept an EpiPen on his belt because he could have a severe anaphylactic reaction at any time. I typically don't take cases like his, but since he had come so far and promised not to ever eat anything that gave him a reaction, I agreed.

His test results were not particularly unusual. We saw him twice a day for four days. He reported feeling fine and went back to Wisconsin. I called him a few months later and learned he hadn't had any asthmatic episodes or allergic reactions since. This nice gentleman has visited us a few times in the last three years for back pain and has not had to use his EpiPen. His dad also referred his wife, daughter, and a friend to us for treatment.

In another situation, a friend referred a woman to our clinic. This dear woman had asthma and sinus problems with so much phlegm that she couldn't walk near perfume or smoke without a severe episode. She rarely went to church and almost never could be near smokers. After five treatments, she walked next to a man smoking and nothing happened! A week later, she was in a kitchen that became filled with smoke and nothing happened. Everyone was amazed! She still experienced side effects from other people's perfumes at church, so we concentrated on fixing the remaining problems. Two months later, she was able to stay in church and even went back for an evening recital. **Update: She continues to do well four years since she started treatments.**

Autoimmune Disorders

When people ask me if acupuncture can treat a certain condition I always answer yes! Of course, the degree of relief depends on many different patient variables. Autoimmune problems can be the most challenging, but we can help with these issues beautifully: Hashimotos Disease, Addisons Disease, Rheumatoid Arthritis, Myasthenia Gravis, and Sjogrens Syndrome to name just a few. Some diabetes and skin conditions can be manifestations of an autoimmune disorder.

We also use homeopathy, nutrition, and herbal medicines with these painful conditions. Please read the section on arthritis and thyroid disorders for more information. One of my first patients came with a dreadful diagnosis and prognosis. I knew her boss, who recommended she talk to me. I explained how acupuncture worked and that there were no guarantees. She was in much pain, exhausted all of the time, and could barely work. Her medical doctor told her she needed to use a walker for the rest of her life. She decided to try acupuncture. In a few weeks, she was able to travel by plane. Her daughter could not believe how much healthier her mom looked. This patient comes in a few times a year for treatment but doesn't need or a walker or a wheelchair, and she leads a very busy life. Acupuncture can work on some of the strangest conditions; it's always a treatment option even if you are under the care of another doctor.

Back Pain
(Middle, Low, and Sciatica)

Back pain is the second leading reason Americans miss work. Back pain can gradually develop or happen quite suddenly. Use heat, ice, or over-the-counter pain relievers for a few days. If it doesn't help, I recommend consulting a specialist in this area—the chiropractic physician. I have over thirty years of experience in the field working with some of the top doctors, and I can positively say that chiropractic care works. According to research, simple stretching can also help the pain, except when people are in pain, they are afraid to exercise or stretch.

For those individuals who do not receive relief from those methods, acupuncture is the next modality in place of drugs. Most people try acupuncture as a last resort and that's a shame. In Florida, you do not need a referral from your primary care physician; acupuncture physicians are quite efficient in treating acute conditions. In fact, if you're not bleeding, have a broken bone, or having a stroke or heart attack, acupuncture would be a wonderful place to start.

Acupuncture and Oriental medicine look at back pain as Channel Obstruction due to Trauma, Qi Stagnation, or a Bi Syndrome. The Bladder Channel, along the spine, is the main area we needle using shallow insertion. We may also insert needles on the outside of your ankle and on your hand by your little finger. We always needle your ear.

We usually prescribe homeopathy or herbals for pain and examine your nutritional situation. Sometimes we recommend weight loss, and my office always encourages you to use a mild to moderate exercise program to build up the back muscles, which will help prevent future attacks. For the chronic back pain conditions of stenosis and scoliosis, acupuncture can help with the pain and stiffness. Some patients need monthly visits, and others do fine with three or four visits a year.

Sciatica

Sciatica is a "pain in the butt" and may even travel down your leg(s). Sciatica is located by the acupuncture points on your lower back around your hips. Sciatica is caused for many reasons, such as the common practice of Weekend Warriors, long rides in a plane or a car, the lack of exercise, or injury. The acupuncture points to treat sciatica are on the Bladder Meridian, and the local points can involve bladder and bowel problems. We will ask you about any changes in your digestive systems. Some people have pain all the way down to their little toe, and some have pain that stops at the knee. The pain may occur on the back of the leg, on the outer leg, or the inner thigh. All of your answers help us to find the correct treatment plan and diagnosis.

Bladder and Kidney Symptoms
Urinary Tract Infections and Incontinence
Kidney Stones and Frequent Urination

A recent study showed how acupuncture helps with bladder control. The Kidney and Bladder Meridians are involved here. Amazingly, many women don't tell me they have this problem but only refer to it when bladder control issues are gone or after we fix something else. We have wonderful homeopathic medicines and nutritional support for these symptoms. Urinary Tract Infections (UTIs) respond quite well with acupuncture, herbal remedies, and homeopathy.

I had a patient with visible blood in her urine. She came to see me for a backache and told me she couldn't schedule an appointment with her MD for two weeks. A backache is one symptom of a UTI. We tested her urine and found a raging infection. We proceeded to treat her and sent her home with herbal medicine to take with lots of water and directions that she go to the ER if her symptoms worsened. She returned to my office five days later. We re-tested her urine and the infection was gone. She said the blood diminished until it was gone in three days. We diagnosed her condition as Damp Heat in the Bladder.

Infections can be so mild that you may never know about it, or it can be so severe, you end up in the emergency room. An infection can also raise your blood pressure and give you a headache. This headache comes up the back of your neck to the top of your head. Some people feel feverish; others don't. We use acupuncture, herbals, and homeopathics to treat this infection. We also counsel the patient on hygiene habits.

I recommend patients wash their underwear separately from other family members with hot water and chlorine bleach and dry the clothes in the dryer. E-coli is the most common bacteria and is very hard to get rid of. We can test the urine and always tell the patient to contact their medical doctor if they get worse. However, most are better in three days when we re-test their urine. This Bladder Meridian condition also involves the Heart and Small Intestine Meridians. The best time of day to treat bladder conditions is between three and seven PM although it is not absolutely necessary to perform treatment during this period.

Many women come in with UTIs, but they act as if this is a normal condition. It's common but not normal! Acupuncture physicians can treat UTIs successfully and monitor this condition closely. I had a patient last week that planned to leave the country on vacation. We ran blood and urine tests for another reason, but discovered that she had a "raging" bladder infection but was unbothered by the symptoms. I tracked her down and sent her to a walk-in clinic for treatment. I also prescribed herbals and homeopathics to take with her on vacation.

Kidney stone pain can be treated with acupuncture. Herbals can also help. I always recommend a patient work with their medical doctor during a UTI episode. We can help prevent other occurrences in the future.

I love working with people who have bladder incontinence! Incontinence involves the Kidney, Bladder, Liver, and Spleen Meridians. Usually women don't tell me they suffer from incontinence or frequent urination until these issues have been fixed. We all know people who can tell you where every bathroom is in the mall! Please send them to the nearest acupuncture physician instead—there's help available!

Bell's Palsy

Bell's palsy can occur overnight and be quite painful. It entails sudden weakness to the face with a droopy eye, which is caused by the swelling of the seventh facial nerve. No one is sure how or why Bell's palsy happens except in Oriental medicine. Practitioners of Oriental medicine believe it comes from Wind and Qi Deficiency. We caution people not to sleep under a ceiling fan or let the air conditioning blow on them. We have treated twenty cases in eleven years with reasonably quick results.

Bowel Conditions
(Ulcerative Colitis, Irritable Bowel Syndrome, Diverticulitis, Diarrhea, Colitis, Loose Stools with Gas, Constipation, and Flatulence)

The above conditions have many things in common and one of these can be diarrhea. They are seven entirely different problems in Western medicine, but in Oriental medicine, they are in the same ballpark. Diarrhea is watery or loose stools. This can be caused by something in the diet, a virus, traveling to a different country with contaminated water or food, food intolerance, poor food handling and storage, jittery feelings, sudden fright, upsetting situations, or a plain old flu. Ulcerative colitis is a chronic disease that typically involves blood in the stool with severe pain and weight loss. Irritable bowel syndrome can have bouts of constipation and diarrhea. If pain, mucus, or blood is present, Heat is obstructing the Large Intestine Meridian. Colitis presents with gas and occasional loose stools. Sometimes there is mucus in the stool. When there is constipation, the stools can be hard like marbles. At times, they alternate with diarrhea and constipation.

When we examine and diagnose using Oriental medicine, we ask questions that are strange to some people. I need to know if your stool smells or floats, what color it is, whether your rectum burns before or after you evacuate, and the time of day you evacuate. These questions help us determine the meridians involved so we can better treat you.

Diarrhea with pain means the Liver Meridian is involved or there is Heat in a meridian. A bad odor also means Heat. Without odor, the problem could be Cold in a meridian and a diagnosis of Spleen or Kidney Yang Deficiency. If the stool is followed by blood, the Spleen Meridian is involved. Very dark stools mean Blood Stasis; bright red blood means Damp Heat in the intestines. We always use the AcuSET protocol to treat these problems.

I had a male teenage patient who was a very severe case; however, after treatment, he was able to have a normal life with friends and a job. Similarly, I am working on a patient from out of town right now. We changed his diet and added nutritional support until he could travel to my office for treatment. He could not have made the trip without this help. We know he will have great success and be able to live a normal life.

One dear older woman had been embarrassed many times over the past twenty years until she became our patient. She had to stop and use the side of the road as a "bathroom" more than once. Other times she left a party or work unexpectedly due to soiled clothing. We were able to end all of that for her with the AcuSET treatments. This female patients experience is not as unusual as many people may think:

Have you ever had dinner and five minutes later had to run to the bathroom because you knew you were going to have diarrhea? Have you ever had abdominal cramps that were as bad as labor pains and made you cry? Have you ever been afraid to put anything in your stomach because you knew you would have diarrhea?

Well, I have experienced all of the above and more. It is like having a constant, horrible stomach virus. I have suffered from irritable bowel syndrome on a steady basis for the last eleven-plus years. Prior to that time, I would have occasional bouts of diarrhea, not knowing why or where they came from. They would last from an hour to a day or so, sometimes one or two times a week. I sometimes could go a week or more without any cramps or diarrhea.

In 1998, I still had severe stomach cramps that medication controlled somewhat but did not eliminate. I took a prescription to stop the diarrhea on a daily basis. After the colonoscopy, I was told by the surgeon not to eat any dairy products, red meat, salads, or raw vegetables, anything with any kind of cream sauce or spices, or anything greasy or fried. So, I was very limited in my food choices. I improved somewhat, but still had diarrhea on a regular basis—sometimes daily, sometimes four to five times a week, sometimes up to eight or ten times a day, but seldom fewer than three or four times a day. That continued until I began acupuncture. In all, I have had three colonoscopies, taken up to eight doses of my prescription drug (my limit) a day to stop the diarrhea, and taken medications that did not really help my irritable bowel.

Since I have had the acupuncture sensitivity treatments, I can eat almost anything. To me, that is a major accomplishment after years of worrying about when and/or where the bouts would hit me. I feel better; I'm surely not as tired. I am not stressed about leaving the house because I might have diarrhea, and my insides do not hurt from going to the bathroom all the time.

Another patient just finished her course of treatments. She is a small-business owner that had diarrhea up to ten times a day. This problem occurred without warning and with no known cause. She also had neck and upper back pain. Acupuncture working with the Large Intestine, Spleen, and Stomach Meridians calmed her problem down to only a few episodes a day in a matter of weeks. She will continue with monthly treatments. She says that now she feels wonderful again and is not afraid to leave the house.

Constipation

Not all constipation problems are from food sensitivities; many occur from a lack of adequate fluid intake, fiber, exercise, hypothyroid conditions, drugs, laxative overuse, colon cancer, lack of muscle tone, liver and gallbladder malfunctions, sluggishness, pregnancy, worry, or not eating enough bulk. Oriental medicine explains constipation as Heat in the Large Intestine, Stagnated Qi, or a Dry Large Intestine with Qi deficiency. A Qi Deficient patient doesn't have enough energy (Qi) to push out the stool, and they may feel exhausted after trying. They may even break out in a sweat and suffer from a headache. The condition varies from either an excess or deficiency and is treated differently. The pulse can be rapid and full with a red tongue and yellow fur or red with no coating.

A sluggish bowel is very common. Most people think one bowel movement a day is normal. However, humans are designed to have a smooth, bowel movement after each meal. You can help correct your bowel problems by chewing your food better (your mom was right again!), increasing your fiber intake (see the section on fiber), drinking more water, and exercising more often. Hypothyroidism, low stomach acid, and a "sluggish" liver function can also cause constipation. Adding the mineral magnesium and green drinks (organic grasses and vegetables in powder form) to increase chlorophyll (a GI healer) or vitamin C can help.

We can treat all types of bowel disorders with acupuncture. If a patient comes in with sinus problems and constipation, we schedule him or her for testing with the computerized electrodermal screening equipment and Food and Environmental Sensitivity Assessment. Sinus problems are also covered under the Large Intestine Meridian, which can be treated with diet changes, herbals, and homeopathy. Our goal is to establish a normal pattern.

For example, an elderly gentleman came to see us. His daughter said that he ate a lot of pasta and rarely any fruit. He had not had a bowel movement in seven days, no matter what they did to help it move along. He felt fruit caused him gastric distress although there was no medical confirmation for this. I treated him for the sensitivities to fruit and asked if they were going straight home. His daughter assured me they would. Two hours later, I got a phone call from her. They had decided to stop at a Chinese restaurant for lunch, and he had had four bowel movements before the cookies arrived because of the AcuSET treatment.

Here is a testimonial from a female patient:

I have struggled with a "lazy bowel" since I was six years old. I would go two or three days without a bowel movement.

In my thirties, it wasn't unusual to go three or four days. Over the years, I went to several doctors and specialists. Initially they tried to convince me it was "normal" to go two or three days without a bowl movement. Later they couldn't find anything wrong with me and told me I needed to improve my diet and exercise.

I tried everything, but eventually it got to the point where it would be five, six, then seven days before I would have a bowel movement. No matter what laxatives I took or what I ate, nothing changed. When I finally told my husband-to-be, he made an appointment with Dr. Rusty, which changed my life. Two weeks after I started treatments, I was having BMs once a day. I have more energy and overall felt better than I had in years. I recently looked at a picture taken two days before my wedding (earlier this year). I was shocked to see how vacant my eyes looked. Now, I have a sparkle in my eyes and feel wonderful. I have enough energy to enjoy my life and look forward to my future. I am grateful to Dr. Rusty and the care she puts into helping her patients. —B.H.

In school, they called me "The Constipation Queen" because I enjoy helping these patients because a good bowel movement is so satisfying! Flatulence or gas can be quite painful. A dear out-of-town friend called to ask for my help. He had severe "farting" for a few days. In fact, he called it "near death by farting." There were no bowel movements just gas with pain. He had tried different herbals and over-the-counter remedies with some help. I recommended he increase his fiber and water along with the homeopathic medicines he had purchased. After another day, he was better. He felt tired and weak for a few more days but recovered nicely.

Chemotherapy Adverse Reactions

Two recent studies have shown acupuncture can help with side effects from breast cancer drugs. Acupuncture can even help increase white blood cells. The WHO listed acupuncture as a remedy for the side effects of chemotherapy many years ago. These side effects include nausea, vomiting, dry mouth, night sweats, hot flashes, anxiety, fatigue, and pain. A number of my patients have sought acupuncture treatment during the course of chemo or radiation. The ones who continued with it did quite well. In fact, a few patients didn't even miss work during their chemo or radiation treatments! Cancer patients become very Qi and Yin depleted during the chemotherapy or radiation, so we see them once a week except for the week after the cancer treatment is given. Additionally, we always work with the approval of their MDs.

Chronic Fatigue Syndrome

Chronic fatigue syndrome is an immune dysfunction that occurs after a virus (Epstein Barr). It is also thought to have occurred after the first swine flu vaccination in 1976. Some researchers believe that recent episodes have been triggered by other viruses and vaccines. The syndrome is complicated, hard to diagnose, and costly. Most people with chronic fatigue syndrome have suffered for a while before they were diagnosed. Chronic fatigue syndrome makes it almost impossible to get out of bed, interferes with thinking, and causes headaches, muscle fatigue and aches, sore throats, and joint pain without swelling. Stress makes its symptoms worsen, and those struggling with chronic fatigue syndrome find that handling stress is harder. It affects more women than men. I test and treat these patients with the AcuSET protocol, nutrition, and homeopathy. We have great success especially with recurrent episodes in alleviating symptoms. In Oriental medicine, this is a Bi Syndrome; Qi Deficiency and other patterns are involved.

Common Colds

When someone comes in coughing and sneezing and with a weak voice, we diagnose Lung Qi Deficiency or Wind Cold. If the person has these symptoms and a sore throat, we call it Lung Yin Deficiency or Wind Heat. These conditions are the common cold and flu. We can also treat these problems with acupuncture.

Some people progress to a Wind Heat that includes a sore throat, sometimes with a fever, and yellow mucous from the throat with a cough or the nose. Acupuncture can eliminate these troublesome symptoms. I have stopped a sore throat (for others and myself) in as little as four hours many times. We treat singers and entertainers before they perform to protect and strengthen their throats and vocal cords.

Coughs

In Oriental medicine, coughs are viewed as reverse Lung Qi. Coughs can be dry, phlegm, weak, or harsh, and most coughs come with a "cold," which is called a Wind Cold or a Wind Heat. With Lung Qi Deficiency, a patient can keep the cough a long time after the other symptoms are gone. The diagnosis would also be Damp Phlegm. We treat this with acupuncture, sometimes moxa. We also have cough syrups and tablets made with herbs or homeopathics that work wonderfully without raising blood pressure or causing other adverse side effects. They are also safe for children.

One delightful woman who approached our office was a smoker and coughed all day for ten years. Her lungs were fine, according to her medical doctor. The doctor said there was no cancer or emphysema, but she had a cough left over from a cold. She was given different allergy medicines, but they barely helped.

The cough bothered her, her family, and her coworkers. Her husband could not hear the TV when she was around. She was desperate and decided to try acupuncture after a friend related the story of how we had helped her.

We did the usual MSA and FESA testing and determined that her Lung and Kidney Meridians were in a weakened state. Her Liver Meridian was in excess as was her Stomach Meridian, which also produced phlegm. We proceeded to treat her, and within a few weeks, her coughing subsided a bit. After a month, her coworkers asked her what she was taking for her cough. Six weeks after treatment, she played eighteen holes of golf without coughing. She also quit buying allergy medicine. We continued to see her once a month for a year. I ran into her in the store a few years ago, and she reported she was still not coughing but would like to come in for tune-ups to keep healthy.

Dental Problems
(Gums and Teeth)

I always recommend my patients see their dentist regularly for checkups. We love our dentist who is open and respectful to our alternative way of thinking. I always ask my patients about their teeth and gums as the first stage of digestion starts in the mouth. When we correct the digestion, general health improves. Statin drugs interfere with the nutrient CoQ 10 and this can increase the risk for bleeding gums (among other problems). Natural toothpastes exist that do not contain harmful additives. Improved nutrition, herbals, and homeopathics all have solutions for gum and teeth problems. We have treated toothaches successfully while the patient was waiting for their dental appointment. Acupuncture produces fabulous results for post-dental surgery pain also. The Stomach Meridian is responsible for the mouth and tongue.

Depression

My Oriental medicine psychology book is HUGE! Depression, anxiety, mania, and bipolar conditions are not new. Some of the treatment protocols go back a thousand years. The imbalance of the Liver and Heart Meridian cause depression. Other meridians are affected also. To begin, we complete a Meridian Pattern diagnosis. With acupuncture, diet changes, and nutrition supplementation, we see results within a few weeks. However, many products are available to us for treating the symptoms.

Digestive Problems
(Gastritis, GERD, Indigestion, Belching, Bloating, Nausea, Vomiting, Stomachaches, and Ulcers)

In Oriental medicine, the Stomach and Spleen Meridians transform and transport the food and nutrients. The Stomach Meridian "cooks" the food; the Spleen Meridian separates the "essences" from the food and drink and then transports the pure essences to the Lung and Heart Meridians where they become Qi and Blood.

We try to educate our patients on the correct eating habits. If you came to us with the medical diagnosis of GERD, I may diagnose you with Stomach Yin Deficiency or Stomach Fire. Hiccups after an illness demonstrate a Stomach Qi Deficiency or a reverse flow of Qi in regular hiccups. Flatulence and bloating can come from Food Stagnation with Stagnation of Qi. The Stomach Qi is to flow smoothly, to cook the food, and to disperse the nutrients easily without medication.

Your body was made to do this complex job without outside interference. Many outside factors including infection from the helicobacter-pylori bacteria create ulcers. Nutritional deficiencies in Vitamin A, B6, C, E, copper, or zinc can contribute also. Overeating spicy food can aggravate the ulcer as will over-processed white flour foods. Antacids can do harm too. Checking for allergies or sensitivities has been helpful, especially if the elimination diet is too difficult for most people to follow. In our clinic, we use acupuncture, correct the nutritional deficiencies, and treat with homeopathy.

Nausea can occur right before a headache or a food allergy attack. Nausea can be due to food poisoning, ear infections, stomach flu, low blood sugar, fear, and anxiety. If nausea happens with a SEVERE headache, that can signal an impending stroke or vascular event, so seek emergency help as fast as possible.

Identifying the cause can help you decide what to do at home. If it is chronic, we will determine the cause using Oriental medicine and then treat accordingly. Indigestion can come with nausea or the urge to have a good burp. This again comes from stagnant food and Stomach Qi. We will work to correct and rebalance the meridians.

We have treated patients who just feel queasy after eating to patients who vomit most days. One young woman was very pale, thin, and tired. She vomited daily. She had no emotional problems

and was not bulimic. She had gone through psychological counseling for vomiting and taken many medicines. We tested her and
found many, many food and environmental sensitivities. After one
week of treatment, she was able to keep food down. Three weeks
later, she came in for a treatment and told me that she had eaten at
a restaurant, visited an amusement park, and even ridden a roller
coaster with no problems.

During the writing of this book, I've had two new patients with
strange but similar conditions. They had severe sinus difficulties
but would also vomit almost daily with phlegm. Their lives were
disrupted to the point of not going to meetings or church functions.
In one week, both of them stopped vomiting. In three weeks, they
both looked like different people with better skin color and sparkling
eyes. The Stomach/Spleen Meridian has a direct connection to the
Lung/Large Intestine Meridians, and the L.I. Meridian is in charge
of the sinuses. Again, our bodies are very complex systems.

Here is a testimonial from a patient with a very complicated
condition. She continues to come in for tune-up treatments for
prevention, and these problems have not returned:

> *I was plagued for months with a digestive/elimination
> problem that my gastroenterologist could not treat. He told me
> to write down everything I ate, figure out what foods caused the
> problem, and simply NOT eat them anymore. Then, in March
> 2005, for two days, I felt as if my whole digestive system
> was suffering the consequences of eating the hottest, spiciest
> Mexican food available. Out of desperation, I called Debra
> Gaffney's office and made an appointment for the next day.*
>
> *When I got there, I started reading through the AcuSET
> procedural paperwork that her assistant gave me. I almost*

walked out. I was stunned and overwhelmed with what looked like an impossible bunch of pre- and post-treatment protocols. However, since I was already there, I stayed and went through my first acupuncture treatment with her.

The next morning, the burning sensation in my digestive tract was gone. My bowel activity was completely back to normal. During the six-week treatment process, I realized that I actually tasted food subtleties again. I wasn't bruising the way I used to (for example, if I even thought about running into the coffee table, I would bruise). A podiatrist had told me the plantar fascitis on my right heel would never completely heal and that I would have to wear arch supports for the rest of my life. Suddenly, it was gone and has yet to return.

**UPDATE – She is doing quite well
and returns for monthly sessions.**

We treat so many patients with stomach problems that sometimes I think no one in America is digesting their food correctly. GERD (Gastroesophageal Reflux Disease) is one of the most common diseases in the United States. Some reports say that 44 percent of Americans experience this once a month, 20 percent once a week, and 10 percent daily. The most popular medications have the side effects of headaches, nausea, and diarrhea. More serious side effects such as broken hips and a type of pneumonia also exist. Acupuncture, Oriental medicine, and the correct nutritional supplements can, in most cases, fix the actual problem.

Nothing is more embarrassing than having gas. It doesn't matter if it is upper or lower. Well, maybe it does when the dog gets up and walks out of the room. Both are very unpleasant, and people tend to talk about them. Bloating and stomachaches sometimes occur. However, there is help with all of these symptoms. We call the reversal of Stomach Qi, Stomach Heat.

People have told me that ulcers feel like someone is pinching you from the inside. Sometimes, people with no real symptoms are diagnosed by their MD. Some ulcers are bacteria related, but all ulcers deal with the malfunction of the Stomach Meridians. Vitamin U, which is found in cabbages, will help heal ulcers. Homeopathics and herbal medicines along with the acupuncture treatments can help heal the body.

The most important aspect of healing any stomach condition is helping people learn what to eat and what to avoid. The right way to eat is in a relaxed setting—not watching the news, but enjoying the company of friends and loved ones. In Oriental medicine, they caution against studying while eating. The Spleen Qi works with digestion and learning, and it shouldn't perform two jobs at once.

Dizziness *and* Vertigo

In Oriental medicine, dizziness and vertigo is a type of Wind invasion. Vertigo is a loss of balance and can be caused by an ear infection or hardening of arteries. With dizziness, you may feel the room is moving or that you are swaying. Dizziness can occur with many conditions such as hypertension, low blood sugar, earaches, pregnancy, and low blood pressure with adrenal gland involvement. One of my very first patients came to see me again recently. He developed dizzy spells this summer while on vacation. He immediately sought medical help. Nothing eliminated his dizziness. After a couple of acupuncture treatments in one week, the dizziness stopped and has not returned in the past month.

Earache, Hearing Problems, Deafness and Tinnitus

Normally if someone has an earache, they contact their medical doctor. For others that use acupuncture physicians as their primary health care provider, we treat earaches with acupuncture and homeopathy. I always caution patients to check with their MD if they don't respond quickly, especially if there is a discharge. Many earaches and congestion from the sinus block the Eustachian tube from draining down the back of the throat. Gargling with warm salt water three times a day really helps. Eating a lemon slice with salt on it (quickly) helps to break up the phlegm.

This spring, I had my first earache in twenty-five years. I forgot how much pain they caused. I had many earaches as a child. I took everything that I thought would work, but the pain was still severe. I used the homeopathic eardrops we had in the clinic. In ten minutes—yes, ten minutes—I had NO pain.

Hearing loss is a different matter, which varies depending on the original cause such as nerve damage or injury. Tinnitus is easy to fix on some patients and not easy on others. Tinnitus can be caused by too much aspirin, use of certain antibiotics, and high blood pressure. Tinnitus can originate from the Kidney Meridian or the Liver Meridian. The pitch determines which meridian is involved, and we treat the meridian accordingly.

Eye Problems

An amazing thing happened while I was going to acupuncture school. I no longer needed glasses to read, which I contributed to the acupuncture treatments. After I had been practicing acupuncture for a couple of years, I realized I no longer needed my glasses to work. I went to renew my driver's license and was required to wear my glasses during the eye test. I almost failed! I was greatly upset because I just had my eyes checked three months prior. I took my glasses off and, with my improved vision, proceeded to tell her what the signs around the place said.

I made an appointment to see my eye doctor right away. He and his staff were baffled. My eyesight had improved so much my glasses were not working. He had to lower my prescription two levels down. I was scheduled to see him again in a month. I went back, and my eyes were still better. The only difference was that I received more acupuncture and I changed my nutritional program by working with a company called Biotics and their protocol for eyesight.

We first started using these new products because we wanted to slow the eyesight loss of some patients. The nutrients most recommended are zinc, lutein, beta carotene, vitamin A, zeaxanthin, omega3 EFA, B vitamins, vitamin D, and vitamin E. We also recommend a low glycemic index diet (www.glycemicindex.com). The best foods to eat daily are kale, spinach, Swiss chard, collard greens, spinach, and fish and fish oils. *All* of my patients on this protocol with acupuncture had their sight improve. One current patient's eyesight improved so very much that I still have trouble believing it but I have the report from her baffled doctor. I continue to have great eyesight; I just use my glasses for driving and hunting (I mean shopping).

Facial Pain (and TMJ)

Face pain usually comes from the nerves in the neck. TMJ is quite painful and causes problems with chewing, which can lead to other problems with digestion and nutrition. I had a patient who suffered from this condition for twenty-five years. He could not smile and was miserable all the time. He retired early and barely had a life. I treated him for a few weeks, and he told me that his pain just stopped. I released him from my care then. It was the most dramatic case in my history. However, I've treated other TMJ problems that are moderate to severe with good results. TMJ is classified as Qi Stagnation possibly with Bi Syndrome. There are great homeopathic medicines in our clinic for this pain.

Fibromyalgia

Fibromyalgia has many different painful, uncomfortable symptoms including but not limited to sleep problems; headaches; sensitivities to light, smells, and sound; numbness; tingling feelings in hands and feet; a sense of hopelessness; and depression. There is also an incredible feeling of exhaustion. The pains can be dull, shooting, stabbing, burning, and deep, or the skin can be sensitive to touch. Other symptoms include restless leg syndrome, mood swings, night sweats, shortness of breath, bladder problems, jaw pain, skin rashes, blurred vision, swollen feet, dizziness, cold hands and feet, a fast heartbeat at times, chemical sensitivities, and allergies.

We see many patients with fibromyalgia and have a very high success rate. We may have to treat them with only acupuncture for a couple of weeks if they are in a weakened state. If that's the case, we then do the computerized electrodermal screening and begin the AcuSET treatments. After we have cleared sensitivities to vitamins and minerals, we prescribe the correct nutritional supplements. Most patients are 50 percent better in a few weeks. It's not unusual for them to return to full-time work with a renewed interest in life. One patient went back to college and became an Acupuncture Physician.

Many years ago, I worked for a chiropractic physician in Connecticut. Our office was located near an allergy specialist who would also send patients to our office for care. These patients were almost "bubble people." They could not live any type of normal life and went to great lengths to get well or at least a little better. One day, I stood by the file cabinet and prayed with much emotion, hoping that there was a better way to help these people. They would go on very restrictive diets to the point of eating only one item for four days at a time. One patient could only wear white cotton. One patient could not use electricity.

At that time, a woman was seeing this allergist. It is coincidence that she became my patient years later. Here is her testimonial:

Allergies have ruled my life since puberty. By age thirty-seven, I was fighting fatigue, pain, and truly severe anxiety attacks, one of which kept me hiding under the bed for two days. I became suicidal.

A famous allergy doctor diagnosed the problems and hospitalized me in Zion, Illinois, in an environmentally controlled facility. During the three-week hospitalization, I was detoxed by four days of total fasting and then tested for food and environmental allergies. The testing showed I was able to tolerate eleven foods and had many environmental allergies. I had to avoid fluorescent lighting, natural gas, and all petrol items. I lived on mono-food meals (one of which was steamed onions) in a four-day rotation, wore only cotton, and carried a charcoal mask to avoid environmental fumes. It sounds bad, but I was pain free and had no anxiety attacks.

I was still plagued with times of sudden weakness, and the formaldehyde fumes were lessened but not eliminated. At the age of fifty, a viral infection damaged the left ventricle of my heart, lowered the ejection rate to 29 percent, and caused arrhythmias.

Now a new round of allergies began as side effects to prescription drugs. These allergies manifested as anxiety attacks, arthritis, fibromyalgia, fatigue, weak legs, and many other symptoms. Meanwhile the food and environmental allergies were again a problem.

At age sixty, I began acupuncture with Debra Gaffney. Now, at sixty-six, I have an ejection rate of forty-five percent, use no prescription drugs, am free of pain, fatigue, and anxiety attacks, and am able to enjoy many more foods. I am truly grateful to Debra Gaffney for her knowledge, her skill, and dedication.

**Update: she is doing well and
has referred many people to this clinic.**

A seventy-year-old woman with an endless list of symptoms came to us as a direct referral from a chiropractic physician. She had been diagnosed with fibromyalgia in 1978 and was desperate for something to work. She rarely slept and when she did had strange dreams. She bruised easily, suffered with sinus problems, and had daily headaches. She had pain over her entire body. She broke out in rashes if she took any medicines. She did nothing all day except try to get through her days. She had tried acupuncture in California and felt it had helped.

On testing with the EDS, we found the health of her meridians was very poor. I could barely find a pulse on her, certainly not twelve of them! She wanted to be treated more than the usual twelve visits because her pain level and tiredness was so severe she couldn't do anything anyway. So we saw her three times a week for three months and then once a week with good results. Over time, her symptoms decreased in severity and number, and she was quite pleased.

Headaches—Migraines, Tension, Cluster

Next to digestion and sinus problems, headaches are a very popular reason why people try acupuncture. In Oriental medicine, there are approximately 720 different headaches and 7,200 treatment protocols not including homeopathic, herbals, and nutritional supplements. I find most people respond after we treat their sensitivities and allergies.

We've had patients with daily headaches. One particular lady comes to mind. She was a schoolteacher and quit her job due to the daily migraines. After a few weeks of treatment, she rarely experiences any headaches. She will be able to go back to doing what she loves—teaching. Some headaches are due to hormones and can continue after menopause. Twenty percent of people experience headaches due to tension at work. With all of our headache patients, we try to show them the benefits of exercise and tension-relieving strategies. It must be miserable to spend days every month in a dark quiet room with racking pain in your head. Unfortunately, most headache sufferers don't have the luxury of even doing that.

Hypertension

High blood pressure is so common in people over fifty that it seems natural to be on medication. Family history, obesity, being overweight, stress, anger, and kidney malfunction can contribute to HPB. It is often called the silent killer and for good reason. Deficiencies in nutrients play a part in HPB also. A popular weekly magazine ten years ago featured an article about hypertension being helped with acupuncture. The story recommends twelve visits with an acupuncturist. I actually had patients bring the magazine to me. In Oriental medicine, there are two types of hypertension; one involves the Kidney Meridian as a deficiency, and the other is with the Liver Meridian with an excess. Acupuncture does a quick job regulating blood pressure and helping with the other symptoms. I also use nutrition, herbals, and homeopathy. We modify patients' diets on an individual basis. I encourage my patients to exercise and do calming activities such as Tai Chi, Qi Gong, Yoga, and meditation.

Hypotension

Low blood pressure can indicate adrenal problems and a very stressful life. We perform a simple blood pressure test in our clinic to aid with the diagnosis. We encourage patients to check with their pharmacy for possible overmedicating of hypertension and diuretics drugs. We also supplement the diet with potassium- and protein-rich foods, adrenal support through B complex, minerals, and vitamin C. Some patients may also need minerals.

Infertility

A few great books have been written about acupuncture and infertility. The latest research shows that acupuncture treatment before and after in vitro fertilization (IVF) increases the chance of pregnancy by 65 percent according to a study published in 2008 from England. I have helped thirty-six women become pregnant. A colleague of mine has an even higher number of success stories. All our babies are pretty and smart with an equal dispersion of boys and girls.

The first thing I do when a woman comes for acupuncture is ask that her husband come for treatments and complete a nutritional health assessment questionnaire. In Oriental Medicine, infertility is a combination of patterns. The Kidney, Liver, and/or Spleen Meridians can be out of balance. Statistics show that 40 percent of the time the woman has an infertility problem, 40 percent the man has a problem, and 20 percent of the time, it is both of them. I encourage husband and wife to lose weight, quit eating junk food, exercise, improve their nutritional status, and receive acupuncture. We have about an 80 percent success rate with just those changes. My heart truly aches for those couples that do not get pregnant, and I hope that someday they do achieve this wonderful gift.

Joint Pain
(Knee, Ankle, Elbow, Shoulder, Hip, Tennis Elbow, Tendonitis, Greater Trochanter Bursitis, and Bursitis of Other Joints, Wrist Pain, Finger Pain, and Carpal Tunnel Syndrome)

The Kidney Meridian governs all the joints. The Bi Syndrome involves the joints, Wind, Dampness, Cold, or Heat. Most joint pain is a Bi Syndrome. No matter which joints hurt, we treat the distal points on the back of the neck and the top of the shoulders. The Gallbladder Meridian points help to eliminate Wind. We also treat local points. If an area is too painful to be touched, we can effectively treat the other side or another location, called a distal point. In Oriental medicine, we have a saying, "Don't punish the child. Support the mother." Essential fatty acids (fish oils) work great with joint pain as well as other nutritional supplements. Sometimes we use electro-acupuncture (a low-voltage electrical current, which is not painful) attached to the needles. Additionally, moxa can be used if it is the Cold type.

One interesting patient who is almost seventy loves to dance and bowls regularly. One late night she had to crawl through an opened window after climbing a ladder because she locked her keys in the house. She's lucky that she only hurt her knee. Someone told her acupuncture could help her. After a couple of treatments, she was back to dancing and bowling!

A lovely woman came to see me for pain in her wrists. She was retiring soon and the pain was unmanageable. Her best friend (another lovely person) recommended us after her successful treatments. I had noticed this woman was very short of breath. She confided she had bigger problems than just pain. I used the protocol for lung problems and before she left she was breathing normally. Each time she came in we treated her wrist pain and breathing. After a few weeks she had more color, more energy and lass pain. She wrote a beautiful testimonial which we included on our website. Now Ms W.P. is retired and enjoying her life and her healthier friend Ms. C.M.

Menstrual Problems, PMS

Thousands of books are available on acupuncture and OM for PMS and menstrual problems. Acupuncture is so successful in the treatment of PMS that I have patients who are so symptom free that they only know their periods are coming by looking at the calendar! Acupuncture and OM balance the entire body. The meridians involved with menstruation are the Spleen, Liver, and Kidney Meridians. The diagnosis regularly includes Qi Deficiency and Stagnation.

With severe cases, treatment takes about three cycles. Acupuncture also alleviates cramps quickly. I encourage my patients to come in for a treatment a day or so before their period arrives and definitely during their period if they have pain and/or cramps. We can regulate ovulation also. The usual symptoms of bloating, weight gain, headaches, moodiness, anger, insomnia, crying for no reason, cramps, and constipation can be gone in three months! We also treat nutritional deficiencies and use wonderful herbals and homeopathy. Difficulty with menstruation is one of the easiest problems to resolve. I had one patient that had such severe symptoms she felt that she would lose control of her actions. We had her fixed up in less than three months.

Menopause
(Jing Duan Qian Hou Zhu Sheng)

There are four stages in life. Menopause is just one of them. Menopause slows down the aging process—rather than speeding it up! A very natural process, menopause does not have to be difficult. When menstruation stops, women stop losing vital fluids and are able to hold onto their Qi, Blood, and Jing. The Yin and Yang are doing a dance at this time. Women lose more Yin (cooling) and the Yang (heat) rises, which is the cause of the dryness and hot flashes.

Forty-nine is the average age for this process. However, women actually are more solid and more in charge at this time. Most women start perimenopause ten years before the actual cessation of the flow. Some of my patients were so filled with rage during perimenopause that they needed to be medicated. Using acupuncture and Oriental medicine with herbs, we were able to help them. You don't have to suffer with the insomnia, hot flashes, dryness, memory loss, emotional rollercoaster feeling, weight gain, clots, pain, cramping, nausea, or breast pain. In Asia, women rarely experience problems with menopause. All fourteen meridians are involved with this powerful process. If you have had a surgically induced menopause, we can still help. The meridians' functions are the same.

Neck Pain and Stiff Neck

Have you ever woken up one morning unable to turn your head? Your first thought probably is that you've "slept wrong." A fan may have been blowing on you during the night or you may have become chilled, which is called Qi Stagnation and Blood Statis. Many meridians run up and down your head and neck. All or one may be involved. We usually treat right where it hurts if possible, which brings quick relief in most cases. If you have chronic neck pain or stiffness, you may also have Bi Syndrome. Some liniments and gels are wonderful herbal remedies that effectively clear the Wind, Damp, Cold, or Heat. Watching your posture and exercise can help acute conditions as well as chronic ones. Movement warms up the meridians, tendons, ligaments, and muscles. It also restores mobility to the joints.

Palpations

Palpations can happen for many reasons, such as a heart problem, fear, anxiety, dropping blood sugar, food allergies or sensitivities, and adverse drug reactions. I am treating a patient suffering from moderately severe palpations. She underwent many different tests, treatments, and medicines. She developed this problem after eating foods with citric acid. If you read labels, you will notice that citric acid is in everything. It is even used as a "wash" for meat. We checked this patient for sensitivities and found many. However, after a few AcuSET treatments with particular attention paid to her Heart Meridian, she's experienced a dramatic change. Her condition would be classified as Heart Qi and Yin Deficiency. Palpations are also treated with herbals and calming homeopathic medicines.

Pediatrics

I could write a whole book on children and acupuncture—in fact, I probably will. Twenty-five percent of the patients in my practice are under the age of sixteen. Children with almost all conditions or illnesses respond quickly.

We have even treated colicky babies who are only three days old. They would scream most of the time and be in such pain. They don't want to eat, which can be dangerous. I always treat the breast milk or formula as a sensitivity that's causing the reaction. Earaches and vomiting are frequent problems also. We have even helped kids with a loose tooth or teeth that are only slowly coming in.

We have a kids' room in our clinic. We can treat them with a microcurrent; it looks like a flashlight. They love it. We let them play with books or blocks during the treatment. I have many times sat on the floor with them. We try to use needles at age four. Most children are open to needling with gentle coaxing. I never push or frighten them. We all remember getting a shot when we were little. I want the acupuncture treatments to be a happy experience for them.

Recent research has reported the possible side effects of cough and cold medicines for children. A Centers of Disease Control report shows that during 2004-2005 over 1500 children aged two and under were treated in emergency rooms for overdoses of cough and cold medicines. In the journal *CHEST*, a 2007 Canadian study found asthma developed in children that received antibiotics in their first year of life. We use safe homeopathic medicines from a company used all over the world, and they are very effective.

Postoperative Pain

A study released in 2007 from Duke University using clinical trials in the United States and the United Kingdom found that acupuncture greatly reduced a surgical patient's postoperative pain and the follow-up need from strong opioids to treat their pain. This study was not news to the Chinese! They have been using acupuncture for thousands of years for all types of pain. They also found it was excellent for postsurgical side effects such as itching, dizziness, incontinence, nausea, stomach upsets, loss of appetite, swelling, scar tissue, and scarring. However, we are off to a good start as 39 percent of hospitals are now using acupuncture.

Pregnancy and Labor

If I help a patient with infertility problems become pregnant, will I treat them during the pregnancy? Yes, if they need it. Only four out of thirty-six women needed to come in for treatment during their pregnancy. Two were for morning sickness and one for a headache. I also had one come in to induce her labor with her OBGYN's blessing. Acupuncture can accomplish all the above including backaches. It can also turn a baby if it is in the wrong position. This is a very old protocol and works beautifully. I only treat my patients who become pregnant and refer new patients who are pregnant to a colleague who has lots of experience with pregnancy and acupuncture. In Oriental Medicine, we call the uterus the "fetal palace." Isn't that sweet?

Adverse Radiation Reactions

The World Health Organization (WHO) and the American Medical Association (AMA) have recommended acupuncture for adverse reactions to radiation therapy for at least fifteen years. I have treated patients for these problems and encourage them to tell others undergoing this treatment to seek out acupuncture. Why? It works! They have less downtime and recover quickly. One patient had radiation treatments on his lunch hour and no one at work knew he had cancer. Two other men worked during the whole time without much of a problem. These three are still cancer free after five to nine years. I help them nutritionally also. After they are through with their treatments, I encourage them to change their lifestyles and eating and drinking habits.

Sinus Conditions, Hay Fever, Sneezing, Itchy & Watery Eyes

The Large Intestine Meridian deals with the sinuses and throat. The Lung Meridian works with the lungs (and skin). The Stomach Meridian with the Spleen Meridian makes phlegm. Together they wreak havoc on most Americans four months out of the year. Some people have headaches or facial pain with coughing and sneezing. Odors can cause a painful headache. Sore throats and earaches can also occur. I have patients that have a runny nose when they eat or some who are so congested and dry that their noses bleed.

We treat patients with acupuncture using points on the face, hands, elbow, feet, and knee. For 95 percent of patients with these symptoms, we use AcuSET treatments. We can stop the symptoms from re-occurring in most cases. If you can tolerate it, eat spicy salsa or horseradish. You can put salt on two slices of lemons and eat them quickly. Salt reduces phlegm. During the "allergy" season, take off the clothes you wore outside in the garage. Don't bring them inside the house until they have been washed. You need to shower before you go to bed and wash your hair as this reduces the amount of pollen or allergens around you while you sleep. Change your pillows more frequently. I had an elderly man once who—no kidding—had the same pillow for twenty years. He purchased a new one and his sneezing stopped.

Listen to this testimonial from one of my patients (G.H.C):

"I am now seventy-seven years old and developed allergies in the late 1980s after living in Florida for about seven years. In 1996, I had surgery for a deviated septum and sinus. I then started having heavy mucous and chronic sinusitis infections two to three times a year, which required antibiotic treatments. Through the years, I sought help from various ENT specialists and tried a variety of prescriptions, nasal sprays, and allergy pills, but the problem remained, and I was told there was nothing more that could be done. I was miserable constantly and felt the antibiotics I was required to take to clear the sinusitis could be detrimental to my health. After my wife's urging, I decided to see Debra Gaffney to try the AcuSET procedure/ acupuncture treatments. After nine of the twelve treatments,

I am off the prescription medicines and my mucous problem has significantly improved. I am hoping the improvements continue and the chronic sinusitis infections and mucous will be a thing of the past."

He did not explain that his mucous was very thick with large amounts on a daily basis. His symptoms were so severe that they interrupted his life. I checked with him recently, and he is doing great.

Skin Rashes

Skin rashes are classified as Lung Qi problems and Heat in the Blood. I have treated everything from minor red spots to a young child completely covered with oozing itchy sores. I have had women that wore gloves all day and night due to the bleeding. I have treated people that had rashes with cracked skin due to the chemicals or papers at their jobs. The common denominator was multiple sensitivities or allergies.

A nail tech came to see us last year. Her hands were cracked, dry, and painful. Since her hands were her tools of her trade, she was desperate. We treated her with the AcuSET technique and acupuncture. In two months, she was smoking less and had lost weight. More importantly, her hands had improved to the point her clients weren't asking her what the problem was. In eight months, her hands were completely clear; the cold weather even quit bothering them. She felt healthier than she had in years, her skin glowed, and her eyes were bright. She is now a very satisfied patient!

The most dramatic case involved a child who was four and a half years old when he came to me. Caleb (his name is used with permission) broke out in a rash when he was six months old. His skin was cracked, oozing, seeping, and itched constantly. His parents took him to all available doctors. He was on many medications including steroids. Caleb cried nearly constantly. His dear mom had to rub thick creams on him and the act of rubbing soothed him a little bit. He was the only patient I had to treat more than twenty times for any condition. He had forty treatments over a year's time. We treated him for everything in his entire environment and any food he would ever eat. After twenty visits, Caleb started to have good days. Sores healed up, there was less agony, and fewer new sores appeared. At forty visits, he was in such an improved state we released Caleb from active care with the promise he would return if his condition worsened.

Five years later, his mom came up to me at our local art show. She asked if I remembered her, and I said, "Of course, we spent so much time together." Then she asked if I remembered the young man standing next to her; I said, "No." She said, "This is Caleb." My eyes began to tear and I could hardly speak! His skin was beautiful—no scars and no sores!

I saw Caleb again last year and he's gorgeous! I haven't experience that type of wonderful success with every severe skin case, but enough improvement that I encourage patients to stick with the treatments. Skin takes a very long time to heal and produce new skin. Essential fatty acids (fish oils) and other nutrients help to support the Lung Meridian and clear out the heat in the Blood.

Sprain & Strains

Muscles, tendons, and ligaments can suffer injuries or tears, which can be mild or so severe they need to be surgically repaired. Acupuncture is wonderful for the field of Sports Medicine and is used in sports injury clinics across the world. For example, acupuncture was available at the last Olympics in China. We don't have to needle the injured area but can use points (Distal) away from injured area to move the stagnated Qi and Blood. Some incredible herbal medicines are available in addition to homeopathy and are used in sports medicine clinics in the United States, Europe, and South America.

Stroke

A stroke is called Wind Stoke in Oriental medicine. The sooner someone can receive treatment, the better the outcome. Conventional medicine won't interfere with acupuncture treatment and vice versa. The only problem is that the rehab centers do not allow acupuncture physicians to treat in their facilities. We have treated people up to three years post-stroke. It takes about twenty visits for progress to appear, in most cases. Patience is needed, but the treatment is worth it. We are very careful with herbal and nutritional supplements as most patients are on blood thinners.

My first stroke patient came to me while I was still an intern. He was in a wheelchair, could not stand up without aid, and could not dress himself. After twenty visits, he could walk in the clinic on his own (with a cane) and could dress himself. He planned to visit Europe with family and friends and made the trip just fine.

Another patient was able to receive treatment six weeks after his stroke. I see him in the grocery store occasionally, and it warms my heart. I inherited another stroke patient from an acupuncture physician that moved away. This man had a stroke in 1995. Apparently, he was paralyzed on his left side. He received treatments from the first acupuncturist and gained much of his independence back. He still comes in monthly. We have seen him gain much strength and mobility as time goes on. It is incredible. He has his setbacks, but he always makes progress.

PLEASE if you know someone that has had a stroke, please make sure he/she visits an acupuncture physician.

Thyroid Conditions

The thyroid gland helps regulate most of the metabolic processes in our bodies. If it is underproductive or over-productive, it will affect your emotions, bowels, skin, sleep, fertility, weight, muscles, menstrual periods, sleep, heart rate, hair, and skin. Your blood work may be normal, but you still have symptoms. This is a common occurrence in most doctor offices and is frustrating for the patient and doctor.

It is estimated over twenty million people have some sort of thyroid condition, mostly an underproductive thyroid also known as hypothyroidism. Acupuncture and Oriental medicine restore the immune function and balance the release of thyroid hormones. Acupuncture can also restore energy, help the emotions, promote normal sleep patterns, and balance the menstrual cycle. In addition, weight loss can be expected. Iodine is by far the most needed mineral for thyroid problems along with calcium, selenium, and magnesium. All these minerals (except iodine) can be found in Brazil nuts and walnuts. Look at the bibliography to find my favorite author on thyroid issues.

One patient in her fifties came in with hypothyroidism, high cholesterol levels, and many other "average" health problems. She was discouraged with the medical route and wanted to try acupuncture.

I explained she also needed a healthier lifestyle. She followed our plan, and in a few months, her lab results were beautiful! She looks more alive and is much more active. She giggled and smiled during the last treatment, which is a change from being so exhausted in the morning that she would plan when she could take her first nap!

Weight Loss

Acupuncture has been popular for weight loss in America since the 1980s. People initially received staples in their ears to reduce appetite, but that practice fell out of favor. Weight loss entails much more than just suppressing the appetite. For example, acupuncture strengthens the Spleen and Stomach Meridians. It gives you more energy in addition to reducing your appetite and changing your taste buds. The *International Journal of Obesity* published a review of thirty-one studies on the treatment of obesity, which included 3,013 people. The study reflected positively on acupuncture and can be found at www.acufinder.com.

We use acupuncture with meal plans, positive mental outlooks, exercise plans, good nutrition, and counseling. We encourage people to focus on what they want in health and how they want to look. We encourage them to have an attitude of willingness instead of worrying about willpower.

I believe the number one problem in America is obesity and excess weight in children and adults. This problem is not getting better in spite of the availability of weight loss information, gyms, workout centers, books, better labeling on foods, etc. Excess weight leads to many physical problems. I work with patients for this condition daily. Acupuncture and Oriental medicine does help with losing weight and keeping it off, but people need to do their part also. To lose weight, you must burn more calories than you put in your mouth. The next step entails working on the emotional reasons for overeating. When I ask my patients why they overeat, the first thing they tell me is they don't overeat—ever.

When I ask them if they exercise, most tell me they walk. They tell me they rarely eat out; they eat many vegetables and drink eight glasses of water a day. Now I know they are telling the truth, but something doesn't add up. I've been overweight in the past, and I know how I got that way, how I got rid of the excess weight, and how to keep it off. In my daily routine, I'd rather spend money on quality food, workout routines, and nutritional supplements than visiting doctors and taking prescription pills. I have my comfort food just like everyone else but in moderation. I prepare ninety percent of our food, and I have the same twenty-four hours a day to get everything done as everyone else. I also save money by not eating out as much or buying processed food. Our daily diet is five to seven servings of vegetables, two servings of fruit, three servings of high quality protein, two dairy servings, three servings of butter or oil, two servings of grain a day with two serving of nuts and seeds and one serving of legumes. We are rarely hungry, and after a day at my clinic, I work out, clean the house, or attend a class, and always go to bed by 10:30 PM.

You can do it too. Motivation is the key. When people tell me that they eat junk food at night, I ask them who bought it, especially with kids. I've never seen a five year old in the grocery store writing a check for cookies and soda. Don't buy it and you won't eat it. We need the willingness to look at what we do to ourselves and to change.

I am not including a meal plan in this book other than the guidelines I've described above. Everyone is different. I like to create a meal plan specifically for each individual, taking into consideration your daily life, habits, and favorite foods.

Water is calorie free and fat free and has minerals—drink lots of it. Decrease your intake of table salt (see the section on salt). Don't use food to handle stress or reward yourself. Take up a hobby that implements your hands. Use purple or blue dishes. Only a few foods in nature are blue and purple (and they are excellent for you), but eating from blue or purple plates is not as appetizing as other colors. Red stimulates the appetite. I know this trick works as I do it.

Walk as much as possible. Use smaller plates, or use your salad plate for your dinner and your dinner plate for your salad. Eat your salad first. Relish what you are eating. A cookie can be four bites—enjoy it and stop. Don't eat cereals. Read labels. Check the fat and sodium contents. Fat-free foods sound like such a great idea, but they contain more sugar and salt. You can have anything for breakfast including a turkey sandwich or leftovers from the night before. Snack on vegetables. I cut them up on Sunday and put them in little containers, so the veggies are ready to grab at a moment's notice. I make a dip with low-fat yogurt and herbs (dill goes well with garlic) or I mix spicy salsa with the yogurt. Get enough sleep and MOVE!

Some people may think I am heartless or don't understand, but I do—I REALLY do. And I feel I have some great tools to offer. These tools are nothing new; there are many programs, books, and diets, but acupuncture does seem to help. I have patients who change nothing else and yet still lose weight with acupuncture treatments. With the AcuSET treatments, we see even better results.

Chapter 7

Nutrition

"Let thy food be thy medicine." —Hippocrates (431 BC)

Every second, we are renewing our bodies. Over fifty trillion cells are constantly changing from birth to death. Every time we eat, breathe, sleep, move, shower, dry ourselves off, rub ourselves, take vitamins or medicines, and exercise, we are affecting our cells. We can affect the process in a positive way by making better choices in what we eat and drink. We can also help our cells by exercising and not smoking or taking unnecessary drugs. If you need to take prescription or the occasional over-the-counter medicines, then you need to learn how to help your body rid itself of possible negative side effects.

We do have some control over our bodies and health or the lack of it. It is not "natural" for people to be on three or four prescription medicines at age fifty or to have a medicine chest filled with over-the-counter pills. It is not "natural" to forego exercise due to pain or tiredness. However, those are common things today.

In the past, the accepted thought by medical doctors was that "vitamin pills" were not necessary. This practice may have been true when our food was grown in healthy soil and went from the field to our table in a very short time. However, now our foods are processed, fertilized with artificial nutrients, sprayed with pesticides, picked green, and then shipped to stores across the country.

If you are in that small group of people who eat five to seven servings of vegetables and two servings of fruit a day, then you are getting a sufficient amount of fiber. Getting fiber is a good thing as we need thirty grams a day for optimal health. But what about the nutrients to support our hectic, stress-filled lifestyles?

If you can't grow your own organic food or buy it from a local market, then buy frozen fruits and vegetables. Frozen veggies and fruits are picked at the correct stage and processed quickly. When you cut an apple or juice carrots and they turn brown, you have just witnessed oxidation and a loss of vitamins. When you cut or tear your citrus, it loses its Vitamin C. Blanching, a quick immersion of veggies in boiling water for three minutes, kills a third to half of the Vitamin B complex and Vitamin C. If you squeeze oranges for juice, the Vitamin C dissipates in a very short time. In these cases, you should use supplements.

Grocery stores are trying to accommodate the growing demand for organic foods and can supply us with more and more variety. Be sure to let them know you appreciate their efforts and help to educate them. There are many more minerals and vitamins that need to be included in your daily diet than I can include here. As you read through the following pages, think about how many food items you eat on a daily basis. What symptoms do you have? If you demonstrated sensitivity to a certain vitamin or mineral, check with us before you continue taking your supplements.

Supplements

Vitamin supplements are insurance policies. In a perfect world, we would receive all of our vitamins and minerals from our food, but that is not the case in our world today. If we could put all the needed daily nutrients into one tablet, it would weigh a pound. People ask why I am so interested in nutrition, and I respond honestly. I see better changes in health when we supplement the missing nutrients. I spend quite a bit of my free time studying nutrition—not how to sell vitamins. Also I don't expect that you'll see your acupuncture physician every day for the rest of your life (it's also not needed), but you need certain nutrients daily. We have a detailed nutritional questionnaire based on your symptoms for you to fill out. In our experience, over a year's time, your symptoms disappear.

Every day, you need to replenish all the B, C, A, D, E, and K vitamins, minerals, amino acids, essential fatty acids, and cofactors. You need these nutrients because there are so many different actions that utilize them in the body to keep you healthy. If you are not producing the correct amount of enzymes for digestion, you are not receiving the vital, life-sustaining ingredients from the food or supplements. Without them, you create degenerative diseases and poor health.

Committees from across the world devised our nutritional daily requirement for nutrients. Their job was to develop a percentage of a particular vitamin or mineral that would help to prevent disease such as beriberi, rickets, and pellagra. We never hear of beriberi or pellagra in this country, but there are reports of rickets among inner-city children.

Rickets is preventable by adequate Vitamin D. Drinking milk with added Vitamin D and fifteen minutes of daily sun exposure would stop this disease according to experts just four years ago. Now even medical doctors are recommending 5000 units of Vitamin D a day. Milk consumption is down across the nation, and soda consumption is up. To save money and time, schools have cut back on physical education, and kids just don't go outside and play the way they used to. Therefore, some are not receiving adequate sunlight. In the defense of our local elementary schools, they are trying to limit the soda served. But does that stop the amount of soda most kids get at home? According to the amount of poor physical and dental health in this country, it does not.

Many people exhibit the signs of nutritional deficiencies: low energy, sleep problems, and a general sense that something is not right. Advertising tells us it is OK to have stomach, sleep, elimination, and pain problems. It's not OK! I see those symptoms marked on ninety percent of my new-patient questionnaires. People feel these problems are "normal." That's the *scary* part; we expect to feel bad, but that's NOT how it has to be. It is possible to wake up ready to start your day without health problems. It is possible to go through your day and get to bed, ready for another good night of sleep.

Homework: Bring in your supplements and your acupuncture physician will go over them with you. You will be able to eliminate some and possibly add others. More importantly, you will be advised on the quality of your supplements. Why waste money on inferior products? Bring in any questions regarding products you have heard about. We can help!

The amount and type of supplement you need may not be the same as your spouse or friend needs. We have different needs at different times in our life. For instance, the average woman's shoe size is eight. Look at your own shoes. Maybe you wear down the inside of your shoe and your friend wears down the outside. Maybe you put more weight on the toes than she does. Maybe you scuff yours on the heels and she doesn't. You both wear the same size, right? You both need the same amount and type of supplements, right? *NO!*

Created in the 1940s, guidelines called recommended dietary allowances, or RDAs, exist for the vitamins you need on a daily basis. In the 1990s, they were updated, and new labeling guidelines (see the section on label reading) were established. This process has helped us become more aware of what we eat, but has confused most people. There are still flaws with these methods because they don't take into consideration how we over-process food, cook our food, and the poor quality of our soil for growing food. It does not take into consideration the different needs of different people. If we compared two women who are the same age, height, and weight with the same jobs and marital status, you wouldn't have the same woman ... just two women with similarities. They would not have the same DNA or RNA. They could have different genetic backgrounds. They could have different health histories and experiences. One may need more protein and one may need less. One may need to eat six times a day and one may do better eating eight small meals a day. So why would a cookie-cutter vitamin pill be all they need?

If you are sensitive to certain vitamins, minerals, or added ingredients in your products, your body will not handle them as well.

One of the possible effects of your sensitivity is the body's inability to absorb and use them. Many of my patients have found after their AcuSET treatments that they were able to use less products or amounts. The idea behind supplementing vitamins and minerals is just not to avoid deficiencies, but to produce optimum health.

In the mid 1990s, a new Food Pyramid was introduced to get us to eat the right amount of foods daily. It is a great idea, but this pyramid really hasn't accomplished its goal, which is evidenced by the number of unhealthy people today vs. twenty years ago. The obesity numbers have increased as well. This pyramid recommends eating six to eleven servings of bread, rice, pasta, or cereal. A serving is one slice of bread; a serving of cereal is a very small bowl. Most people eat three servings of cereal at breakfast without knowing what a serving size is. A typical meal of pasta at your favorite restaurant is six cups, hardly a serving. Who do you know that eats five to nine servings of fruits and vegetables a day? Only 8 percent of the population eats the correct amount on a daily basis. And I am not counting iceberg lettuce and applesauce!

French fries are the favorite vegetable with corn following as a close second. However, French fries and corn compared to other veggies have very low nutritional value, and I don't count them as a vegetable serving. Does anyone really eat the squash and broccoli that comes with your meal in a restaurant? Squash and broccoli are loaded with wonderful healthy nutrients.

Pasta, rice, cereal, and breads are refined and over-processed. They have a shelf life of one to two years. When you eat these foods, they turn to sugar and cause insulin to increase. You want your body to manufacture the correct amount of hormones, not artificially raise them. Some experts think grains cause inflammation in the body. Some of my patients and I have eliminated all grains for six weeks and felt better with an increase in energy and reduction in weight. If you eat whole-grain pastas, breads, or cereals and brown rice, I would only recommend two to three servings a day.

Sugar is hidden in many foods, including salad dressings, pickle relish, ketchup, mayonnaise, peanut butter, and juices. I've even seen it listed in salt! The white flour used in breads, cakes, crackers, and pasta turns into sugar. We have had kids come into the clinic screaming, running around, punching each other, and biting. I'll ask them what they ate that day, and I can count on them saying they had pizza and cake at lunch. No child like this has ever said that he or she had chicken and broccoli that day!

Not all supplements are made the same. I spend so much of my spare time researching vitamins and companies. I've purchased them from TV specials, mail-order companies, catalog companies, old companies, and new companies. I have attended classes and sales pitches for everything that comes along. I have had patients give me bottles to try because they are now selling them to all their friends and relatives. I have also thrown away supplements when I found they did not live up to my strict expectations. There is an inquiry by the FDA right now against seventy-six companies for having lead in their products. I check my facts, and I demand a lot from the companies I use. I have not hesitated to throw out thousands of dollars in products that I found to be inferior. I take supplements, not junk, and I certainly would not prescribe them to my patients. You can always feel safe with the products you find in my clinic, and I hope other acupuncture physicians are as diligent. Acupuncture physicians have wonderful nutritional education, and there are plenty of postgraduate classes to keep us well informed.

Are supplements expensive? No, but they are not cheap either. Being healthy is not cheap. You can buy sixty-four ounces of soda for under a dollar, and all you get is sugar that gives you a quick rush and lets you tumble down an hour later! Your favorite coffee is now two dollars a cup. If you're buying three cups of coffee a week each month, for the same amount you could buy two bottles of a multiple vitamin and a Vitamin B complex in our clinic—more than a month's worth of superior nutrients. Many more, necessary minerals exist and are available in our food (good quality food). Some people need supplementation, and your acupuncture physician can help decide what you need. Please refer to the back of this book for sources of nutritional information. Be careful what you hear on TV, the Internet, or sale brochures. A great many knowledgeable people are out there, but just as many have dollar signs in their eyes.

I ask my patients to bring in all of their supplements, and when they do, I can tell you which patients have insomnia. Do you ever wonder why those products are sold during the night? Aren't you supposed to be asleep—and wouldn't you love to sleep all night? We can help you achieve that and much more. Will you be taking "tons" of vitamins forever? No, that is not our plan. You will take some, and when you run out, you will come by to get more—because you will see the difference in yourself.

In supplementing your diet with vitamins and minerals, look for companies that use whole foods to obtain the vitamin and minerals. In nature, there are complete sources of many small doses of compounds that most of us are unfamiliar with called phyto-nutrients. This group includes phenols, ligans, limonoids, sulforaphane, antothcyannins, carotenoids, reserveratrol, and allicin.

The phyto-nutrients help fight inflammation, regulate glands, make you feel full when you've had enough to eat, and help the organs to work more efficiently. For these reasons, eating whole foods is important. Due to the over-processed diet for most Americans, people do not receive anywhere near the needed amount of these nutrients. Nature knows how to take care of her own. Phyto-nutrients are found mostly in fruits and vegetables.

Vitamin A

Vitamin A is essential for the tissues in the corneas, gastrointestinal tract lining, urinary tract, bladder, lungs, and skin. If you do not have enough Vitamin A, you can develop night blindness, eye inflammations, dry patches on the eyes, reduced resistance to infections, anorexia, crooked teeth, and poor bone and teeth formation. A common sign of Vitamin A deficiency is follicular keratosis. Keratin (insoluble sulfur-containing proteins found in hair and skin) accumulates around the hair follicles and show up on the arms and legs as hard goose bumps, usually gray in color.

Good sources of Vitamin A are whole milk, yellow and orange vegetables, dark green vegetables, carrots, pumpkins, broccoli, squash, collards/mustard greens, kale, dark green lettuce, peppers, spinach, apricots, cantaloupes, and peaches.

Beta Carotene is a precursor to Vitamin A and is a separate component to Vitamin A. It is in the orange, red, and yellow fruits and vegetables along with other components of Vitamin A.

Vitamin A is not flushed out with your urine, so some nutritionists are concerned about toxicity. However, this is rare; deficiencies are more common as you can see by the list of symptoms. In Oriental medicine, it supplements the Blood, fills the essences, brightens the eyes, and clears heat from the Blood.

Vitamin B Complex
Vitamin B1 (Thiamin)

Vitamin B1 (Thiamin) is used to convert amino acids, fats, and carbohydrates to energy in our cells. A diet high in poor carbohydrates, alcohol, saturated fats, sugars, and fast foods accompanied by constant dieting and fasting will provide inadequate Vitamin B complex. No matter how we live or what we eat or don't eat, our need for Vitamin B complex never changes. Without it, we can experience fatigue, anorexia, digestive problems, weakness, muscle tenderness, enlarged heart, slow pulse rate, memory loss, confusion, inability to focus, constipation, nervous system problems (tingling, neuropathy, loss of feeling), and a reduced production of hydrochloric acid. Vitamin B1 clears the Liver Meridian, corrects the movement of the Qi, fortifies the Spleen and Stomach Meridians, dries dampness, and stops pain.

Alcohol can cause Vitamin B1 deficiency, and Vitamin B1 is necessary for alcohol metabolism. So, the very thing you need to process alcohol out of your body is reduced by alcohol. Good sources are pork, beef, enriched cereal, whole wheat, nuts, peas and beans (legumes), milk, spinach, avocados, and cantaloupes.

Vitamin B2 (Riboflavin)

Vitamin B2 helps cells to produce energy. It works with the other B vitamins. They all depend on each other. Deficiencies can cause cracks around the corners of the mouth, inflamed tissues in the mouth, red or tired eyes, burning, itchy eyes, and light sensitivity. It also causes digestive problems as well as malformed and retarded growth in children. Deficiencies also affect our emotions, causing depression and hysteria.

Good sources for B2 are milk, cheese, yogurt, eggs, meat, dark leafy green vegetables, broccoli, avocados, Brussels sprouts, quinoa, tuna, and salmon. Vitamin B2 nourishes the liver, supports the Kidney and Stomach Meridians, and creates fluids.

Vitamin B3
(Niacin, Nicotinic Acid, Niacinamide)

Vitamin B3 has different names. Don't confuse nicotinic acid with the dangerous byproduct of tobacco. Vitamin B3 helps prevent pellagra, metabolizes proteins, sugars, and fats, helps with circulation, feeds nervous system tissue, reduces the harmful cholesterol (LDL), and raises the good cholesterol (HDL).

People with low levels of Vitamin B3 could experience loss of appetite, anorexia, indigestion, bad breath, mouth sores, asthmatic breathing, sleeping problems, headaches, muscle aches and pains, memory problems, and irritability.

Good sources are proteins, organ meat, milk, eggs, chicken, legumes, peanuts, and muscle meats. Vitamin B3 soothes the Liver, harmonizes the Stomach, fortifies the Spleen, clears Heat from the Stomach (a common American problem), and helps Qi to move freely.

Vitamin B5 (Pantothenic Acid)

Vitamin B5 helps cells release energy from proteins, fats, and carbohydrates. It also helps the body utilize other vitamins and increases our resistance to all types of stress by supporting our adrenal glands in the production of cortisone. Vitamin B5 clears Heat, empties the Liver, harmonizes the Stomach, and supplements the Spleen. It helps with fighting infections and with growth. It also utilizes Vitamin D to help our bodies make glycogen and fatty acids (important fuels our bodies need). Vitamin B5 also helps us make estrogen and testosterone.

Neurotransmitter chemicals move information in our brain to our nerves, so if you become deficient in Vitamin B5, you will become tired, feel depressed, experience numbness and tingling in your hands and feet, and develop skin rashes as well as digestive and heart problems. An unusual sign of deficiency is prematurely gray hair.

Good sources are liver and other organ meats, fish, chicken, eggs, cheese, whole-grain cereals and breads, avocados, cauliflower, green peas, dried beans, nuts, dates, and sweet potatoes.

Vitamin B6 (Pyridoxine)

Vitamin B6 is needed in protein metabolism and helps in the making of amino acids (the building blocks of protein). It is used to convert glycogen (muscle energy supply) to glucose, which helps our brains function. It is a natural diuretic and reduces muscle spasms, stiffness in hands, and nausea. Vitamin B6 is important for normal function and growth of red blood cells. People on high-protein diets need to supplement with B6. If you experience carpal tunnel pain, joint pains, burning or tingling in your hands and legs, or sensitivity to light and noise, you could be deficient in Vitamin B6. An unusual symptom is not remembering your dreams. High levels of homocysteine in the blood affect the cardiovascular system. Adding B6 with folic acid and B12 can help.

Good sources are soybeans, legumes, peanuts, walnuts, bananas, avocados, cabbage, cauliflower, potatoes, meat, chicken, fish, egg yolks, prunes, and whole-grain cereals and breads. It clears Heat from the Stomach and Damp Heat from the Gallbladder and harmonizes the Liver and Stomach. It also moves Qi.

Vitamin B12 (Cobalamin)

Vitamin B12 works with amino acids during protein formation and is very important for carbohydrate, protein, and fat metabolism. It works with the brain, nerve tissue, and nerve transmission and is required for red blood cell production. This is the most frequently deficient vitamin in the country. You may have heard of people who needed Vitamin B12 injections. B12 can help with depression, chronic fatigue syndrome, sleep disorders, and multiple sclerosis.

Severe deficiency of Vitamin B12 causes pernicious anemia. Other symptoms can be loss of appetite, tiredness, dizziness, numbness and tingling, confusion and irritability, poor memory, hallucinations, and an elevated homocysteine level in your blood. Our needs for B12 increase if we are pregnant, are over sixty-five, or have hyperthyroidism. An enzyme deficiency can cause digestion problems, and this can create havoc with your production of Vitamin B12. A severe deficiency can cause degeneration of the spinal cord and nerves as well as brain damage. It is depleted by hypothyroidism and lactose allergies. It supplements the Qi and Blood.

Vitamin B12 differs from other B vitamins because it is not found in plants. It is produced by bacteria in the digestive tract of animals and humans or by microbial fermentation of foods. People at risk for vitamin deficiency are vegans, vegetarians (without added sources of B12) smokers, patients with gastric surgeries, and those that regularly overuse antacids, antibiotic use, and some prescription medicines. Microwave cooking can destroy Vitamin B12. This list covers just about all Americans in one way or another.

Good sources are organ meats, clams, oysters, salmon, sardines, egg yolks, and nonfat dry milk. We also get it from fermented soybeans. *An interesting fact:* Vitamin B12 is lost when we grill meat.

Biotin

Biotin works with the metabolism of proteins, fats, and carbohydrates. It helps folic acid to do its job better. Biotin produces healthy hair. Deficiencies can result in skin rashes, anemia, anorexia, nausea, and muscle pain.

Good sources are liver, organ meats, molasses, and milk. It nourishes the Blood, supplements the Heart, and quiets the Qi.

Choline and Inositol

Choline and Inositol are other components to the B complex. A good formula has all of the above listed on the bottle and in the tablets or capsules.

Choline works with Inositol to form a basic ingredient in lecithin, which can be found in egg yolks, liver, and wheat germ. Choline helps with the covering of our nerves, regulates liver and gallbladder functions, and prevents gallstones. It is also helpful with hypertension and cirrhosis of the liver. Inositol is found in the spinal cord nerves. It protects the liver and arteries and is needed for brain growth and cerebrospinal fluid. High doses of Inositol can help with pesticide poisoning and nerve pain.

In Oriental medicine, Inositol and Choline nourish the blood, moisten the intestines, supplement the Liver and Kidneys, help with the free flow of bowel movements, and extinguish the tendons, ligaments, and bones. They also quiet the spirit.

Folic Acid

Folic acid is one of the most common deficiencies in America today. Most of it is lost in cooking and food storage. Many medicines interfere with the absorption and metabolism of folic acid. If you experience any of the following symptoms, you too could be deficient: headaches, memory loss, weakness, diarrhea, digestive problems, weight loss, irritability, sore tongue, and palpitations.

Homocysteine levels that are low can be raised with folic acid. During pregnancy, a certain type of anemia can develop. Folic acid also quiets the spirit and the fetus. Birth control pills also reduce folic acid absorption, which is such a serious problem that the food industry is adding folic acid to orange juice.

Good sources are dark green veggies (folic = foliage), organ meats, kidney beans, asparagus, broccoli, beets, cabbage, cauliflower, orange juice, cantaloupe, green peas, legumes, sweet potatoes, wheat germ, and whole-grain cereals and breads. It nourishes the Blood and harmonizes the Liver.

Vitamin C

Everyone knows oranges contain Vitamin C. But most people don't know that Vitamin C is lost a short time after the orange is cut. Light, heat, and chemicals also destroy Vitamin C.

Vitamin C helps us make collagen, an important protein that binds muscle cells together. It is found in bones, teeth, skin, and scar tissue. Vitamin C helps prevent bruising, works with cholesterol metabolism, and aids folic acid and iron absorption. Since Vitamin C is destroyed by heat, light, and air, we usually need to supplement with capsules. Vitamin C is considered an antioxidant. Antioxidants slow down the aging process in our bodies and work with our cells in hundreds of processes. Vitamin C helps our bodies with the detoxification process of lead, excess copper, iron, bromide, arsenic, and pesticides and reduces the effects of cancer-causing agents.

If you are deficient in Vitamin C, you may experience anemia, bleeding gums, bruises, loose teeth, sores in your mouth, joint pain and tenderness, chronic constipation, slow wound healing, frequent colds, and/or allergy symptoms. If you are under stress—physical or mental—your need for Vitamin C goes up.

Good sources are citrus, tomatoes, green peppers, parsley, dark green leafy vegetables, broccoli, cauliflower, strawberries, cabbage, potatoes, and green peas. It clears Heat and resolves Toxins.

Vitamin D

Vitamin D helps with calcium absorption from the intestines and re-absorption from the bones. Vitamin D also works with the body's excretion of calcium and moves calcium and phosphorous to the bones and teeth. It acts as both a vitamin and a hormone. It is produced in human skin and is activated by the sun's ultra-violet rays.

Vitamin D deficiencies produce rickets in children and osteomalacia in adults. It has been shown to increase bone mineral density in people of all ages but especially over age sixty-five. Five years ago, we heard very little about Vitamin D; now it is considered a "miracle vitamin." This is a perfect example of how little we know about the nutrients and their importance in creating and maintaining health. Vitamin D can also help with bipolar disorders, depression, and maybe schizophrenia. On any patient blood test, we find low levels of Vitamin D, even those living in Florida! It also works with insulin production and diabetes. In Europe and Africa, high doses of Vitamin D have been used for the prevention and treatment of the flu. There are no studies that I could find in America, but I did notice that our patients had a lower level of incidences of the flu this past year. Because of its importance, our patients are on Vitamin D supplementation.

Celiac disease (ingestion of gluten found in grains that is not digested correctly and causes chronic mal-absorption syndrome, diarrhea, cramping, fatigue, and weight loss) is affected by Vitamin D because the absorption depends on bile secretion and fat absorption. Vitamin D helps with weight loss, glucose, and insulin metabolism. It is also useful in hypertension. Studies also show that Vitamin D is deficient in people with lupus, multiple sclerosis, rheumatoid arthritis, and Type 1 diabetes.

Good sources are cod liver oil, fish oils, and the edible portion of oily skin on salmon, herring, and sardines. It is also found in fortified milk and cheese. The RDA for Vitamin D has been increased in the last few years.

It is almost impossible for vegetarians to obtain adequate amounts of Vitamin D by diet alone. Thirty minutes of sunlight a day is very helpful. Sunscreen, smog, clothing, fog, and pollution interfere with the absorption of the sun's helpful rays. Vitamin D supplements the Kidneys, invigorates the Yang, strengthens the sinews and bones, and brightens the eyes.

Vitamin E (Alpha, Beta, Gamma, Tocopherol)

Vitamin E protects the lungs against oxidative damage from air pollutants and protects skin tissues, eyes, liver, breasts, and calf muscles. It works to maintain Vitamin A's integrity. Vitamin E is useful for structural and functional maintenance of cardio-, skeletal-, and smooth muscles. Vitamin E aids the red blood cells. A deficiency can cause a miscarriage or re-absorption of the embryo.

Good sources are vegetable and seed oils. Safflower oil is the best. Cooking and food processing reduce Vitamin E. Wheat germ is a good source, but when flour is milled, it loses Vitamin E. In the bleaching process, Vitamin E is destroyed if chloride dioxide is used. Other sources are green leafy vegetables, wheat germ, egg yolks, butter, and nuts. It nourishes the Blood, supplements the Yang, and strengthens the ligaments, tendons, and bones.

Vitamin K

Vitamin K helps the liver's formulation of prothrombin, which starts blood clotting. When you are deficient in Vitamin K, you can hemorrhage or, at the very least, bruise more than normal. Vitamin K needs fats such as bile to be absorbed. Long-term use of blood-thinning drugs will increase the need for Vitamin K. If you are on blood thinners, you need to discuss this with the prescribing physician.

Vitamin K is found in dark green leafy vegetables. Vitamin K works with the lungs and large intestines (astringes) and stops bleeding.

CoQ10 (Ubiquinone)

CoQ 10 is found in every cell. We make our own supply, but it's not enough to combat the daily assault of bad food, lack of vitamin and minerals, and some prescription medicines. Low levels have been associated with chronic fatigue, high blood pressure, heart disease, infertility, and diabetes. CoQ10 decreases with age, stress, alcohol, and smoking also. The best way to get it in your diet is to supplement it. Cholesterol drugs called stains rob the body of CoQ10 because they block the same enzyme that is involved in CoQ10 formation, which can be dangerous.

Minerals

Calcium

The average woman has approximately three pounds of calcium in her body. We have more calcium in our bones than any other mineral. It helps with bone strength, blood clotting, and electrical conduction in the nerves and heart. Calcium needs other minerals, especially magnesium and vitamins (particularly D), to complete the picture. Taking calcium alone will not build stronger bones. Many calcium supplements are available. Calcium citrate is a great source, and calcium carbonate is not.

Good sources of calcium are dark green vegetables, legumes, tuna, sardines, salmon, sesame seeds (although you would need to eat tons!), milk, and yogurt. Calcium is a good mineral to use as a supplement in combination with other minerals to support it. Calcium and magnesium work together with reducing pain, relaxing muscles, and keeping bones strong.

Research shows that a lack of calcium among other minerals causes osteoporosis, osteopenia, eclampsia, and some forms of hypertension. It calms the Yang aspect, the over-energetic part. It astringes Yin and suppresses overexcited Yang. Calcium also absorbs acid and stops pain.

Chromium

Chromium is an important mineral to maintain blood sugar levels. It also works with amino acids with utilization of protein synthesis in addition to hundreds of other functions like all the minerals. In nature, the right combination of minerals, vitamins, amino acids, carbohydrates, and fats are balanced. For these reasons, it is very important to eat a healthy diet and to supplement with whole food tablets or capsules. Chromium is found in wheat germ, bran, whole-wheat bread, oysters, corn meal, whole grains, clams, molasses, and kelp. Chromium fortifies the Spleen, boosts the Qi, and supplements Qi and Blood.

Iodine

People are familiar with iodine and hypothyroid. Iodine also is important for the prevention of mental health, autism, ADD, cholesterol, and cardiovascular disease. Along with other minerals, it helps to treat or prevent asthma, breast, ovary, prostate, thyroid cancer, diabetes, excessive mucus production, hypertension, keloids, liver disease, and preeclampsia.

A large incidence of goiter occurred in people who lived in the upper Midwest. The introduction of iodine into salt in the last century helped reverse the occurrence of goiter, but in the last twenty years, people have added less salt in their diets although there is a large amount of salt in our processed foods. Quite a few studies are available on the Internet regarding iodine. I have barely touched on the subject here, but I do have additional information available for my patients. Iodine is available in seafood, but most of our iodine is added to multiple mineral tablets.

Iodine courses (clears and creates) a good flow of the Liver Qi and strengthens the general overall Qi. It also clears heat.

Iron

Almost everyone has heard that iron is needed for healthy blood and to prevent anemia. Its main job is hemoglobin formation. Iron supplements are needed for women of childbearing age, especially during pregnancy. Some people will need to supplement with iron after surgeries or traumatic injuries that cause blood loss. Some children also need supplementation. Iron deficiencies are discovered through routine blood tests.

Good sources are lean red meat, fish, chicken, citrus fruit, tomatoes, broccoli, pumpkin, cabbage, quinoa, and chickpeas. Most cereals are enriched with iron. It clears Heat and cools the Blood. Iron also quickens the Blood and eliminates stagnation.

Magnesium

Magnesium plays a role in keeping our cells working properly. It is required for the metabolism of most minerals and for the production of hydrochloric acid. It plays a major part with calcium in bone production.

Magnesium-deficiency symptoms include muscle weakness, muscle pain and stiffness, spasms, spastic colon, migraines, tension headaches, eyelid twitches, tremors, irregular heartbeats, anorexia, and depression. It has been associated with hypertension, preeclampsia, diabetic disorders, Reynaud's disease, leg cramps, and heart disease. Many drugs such as diuretics and antibiotics cause you to lose magnesium. On the other hand, large doses of magnesium can cause diarrhea. If you have sluggish bowels or dry stools, increasing magnesium is beneficial.

Good sources are dark green leafy vegetables, quinoa, nuts, and legumes. It suppresses Yang and astringes Yin. It also quiets the spirit and stops pain while relaxing the muscles.

Molybdenum

Molybdenum is one of my new favorites! No matter how I treat myself with AcuSET for the chemicals used in hotels and conference rooms, my eyes still become red and swollen when I attend classes and conferences. These chemicals are irritants and cause lots of problems for living creatures. They are great for killing bacteria and cleaning. My dear friend and nutrition mentor Donna Lannom introduced me to this incredible nutrient, molybdenum. Now I can attend class without looking like I sat up all night crying in my beer! Molybdenum nourishes the Blood, enriches the Yin, clears heat, and cools Blood.

Potassium

Potassium is the main electrolyte in our cells. There is a fine balance in our cells with potassium, sodium, and chloride. In this country, we ingest too much sodium and not enough potassium. Potassium is lost through diuretic and antibiotic use and when food is boiled. Eating foods raw or steamed in moderation is better.

Low levels of potassium affect blood pressure. If you are taking a hypertension drug that also is a diuretic, your prescribing physician will recommend potassium supplementation. Symptoms of deficiency are diarrhea, nausea, muscle weakness, dizziness, flatulence, mood changes, and cardiac arrhythmias.

Good sources are squash, potatoes, spinach, lentils, legumes, peas, raisins, orange juice, cantaloupes, and bananas. Potassium fortifies the Spleen and clears dampness. It clears Heat, dispels Wind, and eliminates Damp Heat.

Selenium

This mineral is needed to prevent premature aging, liver spots, anemia, chronic fatigue, cataracts, high blood pressure, impotence, infertility, PMS, low birth weight, and birth defects. Selenium works with manganese and Vitamins A and E. It is found in Brazil nuts, wheat germ, broccoli, mushrooms, celery, cucumbers, asparagus, garlic, brown rice, whole-wheat grains, onions, tomatoes, and some herbs such as hawthorn, ginseng, and red raspberry. We don't need much on a daily basis, only 60 to 100 mcg.

Selenium astringes Yin and quiets Yang and the spirit. It also brightens the eyes.

Silicon

Silicon—no, not the ingredient in breast implants but a real honest to goodness mineral from the earth! Deficiency signs are sagging or wrinkled skin, dull, thinning hair or hair loss, insomnia, soft brittle nails, osteoporosis, poor bone development, and a slow growth rate.

Silicon supplements the Liver and Kidneys, strengthens the bones, tendons, and ligaments, and does a great job for the skin. Another dear friend and nutrition mentor Joell Daniels introduced me to this marvelous mineral. Silicon is found in whole grains, nuts, seeds, pears, plums, grapes, parsley, asparagus, cabbage, red beets, pumpkin, celery, cauliflower, tomatoes, peas, red peppers, lentils, and soybeans.

Sodium

Sodium is an important mineral. It is involved in the delicate electrolyte balance in our cells. If it gets out of balance, other minerals will also. An imbalance can cause edema, hypertension, heart disease, and kidney disease among other problems. Sodium is available in celery, leeks, onions, parsley, figs, okra, watercress, seafood, and papaya. Celtic salt contains sodium and at least sixteen minerals. Some deficiency signs are vomiting, heat stroke, muscle cramps, weak and sluggish sperm, and infertility. This type of sodium is not to be confused with over-processed sodium chloride that is used in packaged foods (see the next section on salt).

Salt

By salt, I mean the salt derived from sea salt, not the version that is stripped of minerals, bleached with sugar, and bombarded with fillers. We need salt in our diet. Our cells are composed of sodium, potassium, calcium, and magnesium. It is a very delicate balance. Unrefined salt is sea salt and has the balance of the sea. It is easy to find in the local health food and grocery stores, *but* read the label. Some people on high blood pressure medicines are on a restricted salt diet. Please adhere to your medical doctor's orders but also research sea salt. In my experience, nearly none of my high blood pressure patients use salt-free or low-sodium foods.

Salt supplements the Kidneys and Liver, secures the essence, softens hard masses, and dissolves phlegm.

Sulfur

Sulfur is found in protein-containing foods such as fish, clams, peanuts, and Brazil nuts. It is also found in asparagus, garlic, onions, apricots, kale, broccoli, wheat germ, celery, horseradish, and turnips. If someone is deficient, they would show symptoms such as difficulty in thinking, memory loss, sluggishness, skin rashes, hair loss, blemishes, dry flaky skin, and brittle dull nails.

Sulfur supplements the Kidneys, warms the Yang, blackens the hair, and helps the skin. Sulfur is not the same thing as sulfa drugs, which many people are allergic to.

Zinc

Zinc is involved in numerous activities like building cells and their metabolism. It works with DNA creation and cell dividing. The lack of zinc causes sleep problems, sensitivities to foods, and loss of sex drive. Zinc is found in pumpkin seeds, nuts, peas, eggs, whole grains, oats, beef, and oysters. Remember the age-old saying of eating oysters before "a big night"?

Zinc nourishes the Liver and enriches the Kidneys. It also strengthens the bones and brightens the eyes.

Basic Components of Food

Carbohydrates

Ah, carbs! We crave them, stuff ourselves with them, and lie to ourselves about it. Carbohydrates are addictive. Don't believe me? Give up any bread, cereal, cake, cookies, crackers, pie, rice, pasta, and pizza for three weeks. Just the thought sends shivers down the spines of many of my patients. I refused to do it the first time I was challenged.

Then I did it. I noticed after week one that it wasn't too hard; then came week two. That was difficult. I would've given my kingdom for a cracker! I kept on; I had made a promise, and I keep my promises. After week three, I ate a cracker, but it tasted terribly gooey! I was sure I just had a bad cracker so I ate a piece of toast, but that was even worse. It tasted like a ball of dough.

I took an inventory of myself; my hands didn't ache after needling forty-five patients. I slept all night, and I lost five pounds. I suggest a carb-free diet for three weeks to my patients and *always* meet with resistance, which tells me that we are addicted. My most recent patient did do the diet and succeeded but on day twenty-two ate a piece of toast in the morning. Every time she saw me, she talked about toast. She did admit that she was feeling better and lost ten pounds—a very difficult-to-lose ten pounds!

Carbohydrates provide energy, help proteins to metabolize, and provide bulk to assist in digestion, elimination, and absorption. Carbohydrates are necessary to help us fight infections and for the growth of bones, skin, nails, and tendons. Carbohydrates provide glucose for energy for the red blood cells, brain, and central nervous system.

As with fats, there are good and bad carbohydrates. Good ones are found in vegetables, grains, fruits, and legumes. When most people think of carbohydrates, they think of sugar. Sugar is divided into two types—simple and complex. Simple sugars are junk foods: soda, candy, cakes, cookies, syrups, and white sugar. Fruits and vegetables contain complex sugar. This knowledge helps people to understand the difference in carbohydrates and the secret to weight loss for most people.

In the 1970s, a popular diet emerged—limiting carbs to almost nothing. People lost tons of weight but could not sustain this way of eating for too long and so gained it all back. This diet came and went over the next thirty years. It's been modified now but is still too restrictive for most people. In the 1990s, a new system came out. It separated the carbs using the glycemic index. When we eat too many carbs, and most of us do, we gain weight, develop sugar-digesting problems, raise our cholesterol and triglycerides, and put fat on our bodies. Excess carbs are changed with insulin into glycogen, stored in the liver and muscles, and then changed into sugar for a form of energy. It also changes into cholesterol (the bad kind LDL) and into saturated fat (which looks like the fat you cut off a steak); saturated fat becomes triglycerides and is stored in fatty tissue.

Next, we have simple carbs versus complex carbs. Simple carbs break down faster and give our bodies a "rush"; complex ones break down slower and provide energy to our bodies and brains. Simple carbs are mostly junk food and most breads, rice, pasta, and cereals. They leave you tired and with difficulty concentrating or thinking at all. They burn up quickly and then cause a drop in blood sugar. This also causes hyperactivity, anxiety, headaches, sleep problems, panic attacks, depression, anger, frustration, problems with thinking clearly, and making decisions. Is a cookie or some spaghetti worth all of the above?

A life like this (which 85 percent of Americans are living) causes weight gain and degenerative diseases. Degenerative diseases have become so typical that people think this is part of the aging process. Ask yourself, *Why am I a slave to what I put in my mouth?*

The glycemic index is a secret weapon to weight loss and a healthy life. Diabetics have been using it for years. The index measures the amount a food can raise your blood glucose. Glucose is a value of 100; for example, the glycemic index (G.I.) of rice cakes is 78, and for peanuts, it is 14. Eating four ounces of peanuts is better for your brain and blood sugar than a rice cake. A serving of whole-wheat spaghetti (1 cup—I know but try it) has a G.I. of 37, and that's good. Throw in some lean ground meat and a sauce made without additives such as sugar and you have the healthy start of a meal.

For the complete glycemic index and it's huge, go to www.glycemicindex.com. Stick with foods with a glycemic index of 10 to 55.

Lately my patients have been asking about high fructose corn syrup and its dangers. Articles floating out on the web show various pros and cons. Flavored water drinks are everywhere also. I showed one patient how much sugar she was getting from three bottles a day of her fancy water. Athletes that work extremely hard in the hot sun do need additional electrolytes, but the average gym workout does not require anything more than water.

I have never been a fan of fruit juice either. In nature, we would not eat the eight oranges or six apples in a day that a glass of juice contains. Fructose derived from fruit is sugar. Sugar in large quantities causes obesity and diabetes. People need to use less sugar of all kinds—not add it to their water.

Let's face it: Sweet foods or drinks give us pleasure. Breast milk is sweet, and we go downhill from there. We have taste buds on the tip of our tongue that are used only for tasting sweet flavors. I am sure that we are addicted to sweet foods and drinks.

Just try to NOT eat any grains for three weeks. When I ask my patients to do this, they all act as if I've asked them to commit a horrible sin.

Complex carbohydrates are also found in legumes, peas, nuts, whole-grain pasta, quinoa, brown rice, barley, buckwheat, rye, and cereals and have a lower glycemic index.

Enzymes

Almost all enzymes are proteins and are produced in the mouth, stomach, small intestine, and pancreas. Enzymes break down proteins (protease), fats (lipase), carbohydrates (amylase), and milk (lactase). To promote digestion of food into particles for absorption, we also ingest enzymes from our food. There are over 3,000 enzymes, and they aid in almost every action in the body. As we age, we produce fewer enzymes. Enzymes help maintain your immune system, and clearly, we all need more help with this process.

Enzymatic production can be affected by not eating enough raw fruits and vegetables as well as by some medications, illnesses, and traumas. Supplementing your diet with enzymes can produce amazing results in less than two weeks.

Fats

The average diet contains more fat than necessary for optimal health. Fat is essential, and there are good fats. Unfortunately, most people do not know the difference. There is an overabundance of Omega-6 fatty acids in the average American diet, which causes inflammatory diseases such as arthritis and heart disease. Omega-6 fatty acids come from non-organic eggs, vegetable oils, meats, and fish.

The good fatty acids can't be made in the human body and must be added daily to the diet. These Omega-3 fatty acids help the cells communicate with the genes. Good fatty acids are found in seeds, nuts, vegetable oils, and nut and flaxseed oils. Essential fatty acids are also found in coldwater fish, rabbit, and wild game.

Most of the oils used today are processed polyunsaturated oils and are dangerous. These hydrogenated oils are in all processed foods. We know these as trans fats. Science has proven that these fats contribute to common degenerative diseases such as arthritis, diabetes, and obesity. This research has created uproar, and some states have banned the fats from popular fast-food restaurants.

The preferred cooking oils are coconut oil, extra virgin olive oil, sesame oil, and sunflower oil. Use butter and never margarine or the "spreads" that are low in fat or cholesterol.

Fats are essential for making cell membranes and hormone production. Fat acts as a carrier for the fat soluble Vitamins A, D, E, and K. People have been told to keep a low-fat diet, but obesity has increased over 30 percent in the last twenty years. Cholesterol is needed as an important molecule for hormone production. Protein cannot be used without the proper amount of fats. Essential fatty acids are so important that a deficiency can contribute to abnormal clotting, heart attacks, hypertension, strokes, and other conditions such as arthritis, allergies, dry rough skin, psoriasis, brittle nails, hair loss, asthmatic breathing, migraines, and decreased fertility.

Thirty to thirty-five percent of our daily intake needs to be fats, but they must be the correct fats. The correct fats are polyunsaturated fats found in whole foods like fish, fish oils, nuts, seeds, and soybeans. The best sources for mono-saturated fats are found in avocados, almonds and other nuts, and eggs. The bad fats are the trans fats, which are found in processed foods. They alter the normal fat functions. It takes fifty-one days for your body to metabolize trans fats.

Trans fats are formed during a process called hydrogenation. This new substance is bad for our cells; it causes them to leak and distort their shapes. This will promote deficiencies in vitamins and minerals. I try very hard to not eat them. It requires more baking at home to eliminate them from your diet. Read labels! Another term for the bad fats is hydrogenated oils. They are also called hydrogenated vegetable oil, partially hydrogenated cottonseed oil, and hydrogenated soybean oil. They are found in popcorn, cookies, cakes, fast foods, peanut butter, and chips.

Saturated fats are somewhat in the middle and are found in milk, meat, coconut oils, butter, and processed foods. We need the good fats daily, and it's easier to supplement with a source of fish oils. The controversy over fish rages fairly strong right now in the nutrition world. We like to use only two specific companies that can prove to us where the krill or anchovy source came from and the lack of added chemicals.

Fiber

In our Western society, we have more constipation, hemorrhoids, anal fissures, diverticulosis, diverticulitis, gallbladder disease, hiatus hernia, gas/flatulence, obesity, high cholesterol levels, coronary disease, polyps, colon and rectal cancer, and varicose veins than we did forty years ago. In countries with diets high in fiber, these diseases and symptoms are rare.

If you just added legumes (black beans have eight grams of fiber in a half cup), vegetables (peas have five grams of fiber in a half cup), fruit (pears have five grams in one small pear; half of an avocado has eight grams), whole grains (brown rice has three grams of fiber in three-fourths of a cup), barley (thirteen grams of fiber in one cup), buckwheat groats (five grams of fiber in one cup), a slice of whole wheat bread (two grams of fiber), flaxseed, or whole wheat pasta (one cup is six grams of fiber) to your diet, you could change your health dramatically. The average fiber intake is thirteen to seventeen grams a day. It needs to be increased to twenty-five to forty grams a day. Be sure to have adequate water intake to keep things moving along smoothly!

Proteins

Every cell in your body is basically protein in nature. Partially broken-down proteins get into the bloodstream and can cause allergies. Almost 20 percent of our lean body mass is composed of protein.

Amino acids are the building blocks of proteins and contain a usable form of nitrogen. There are twenty types of amino acids. Nine of these, the essential amino acids, must be eaten as food on a daily basis as they are not produced in the bodies of mammals. The other, nonessential, amino acids are produced in the body.

The most complete proteins are from animal sources. Plant proteins lack one or more of the essential amino acids. If you choose to only eat vegetables and grains, you will need to learn to correctly balance your protein intake.

Protein digestion starts with cooking the meat, which softens the connective tissue and makes it easier to chew, swallow, and break down. Next, the stomach takes over, using enzymes and stomach acid to continue the digestion process. Whole proteins are absorbed except when we are under five months old. Infants can't absorb whole proteins in their intestines, and this can create allergies later in life. Cow's milk and egg whites are two of the most common allergens. In adults, less hydrochloric acid and decreased enzyme production will cause gastric upsets.

In Oriental medicine, amino acids fortify the Spleen, supplement the Qi, Yin, Blood, and Yang, clear heat, cool the Blood, quiet the spirit, extinguish wind, and dispel dampness.

Super Oxidase Dismutase (SOD)

SOD is the fifth most common protein in the body. SOD with catalase controls and removes poisons from the body. It is great for anti-aging factors by controlling the free radicals in the body. It works with many different functions in the body such as reducing inflammation, protecting from malignancy, and reducing morning stiffness and joint swelling. SOD is found in barley juice and in certain melons.

Portion Control

The average serving of spaghetti in a restaurant is really five servings. A bagel is really four servings. People rarely eat just fourteen nuts, but that's a serving. One serving of cheese is about the size of the top of your thumb. Those cute little butter pats are one serving. A serving of vegetables on the other hand is about the size of your hands cupped together. A serving of meat, fish, or chicken is about the size of your wallet. A serving of baked potato is the size of your computer mouse. See where we're going here? If you want more food, eat vegetables. For more information, go to www. glycemicindex.com and follow the guidelines for eating foods with a GI value of 10 to 55.

Artificial Sweeteners

I ask my patients many questions. One is the amount of artificial sweeteners they consume on a daily basis. I encourage them to quit and quickly. If you check the Internet on this subject, you will find conflicting information. I know from experience that the patients who quit drinking diet sodas and artificial sweeteners see positive changes in their health.

One patient was scheduled for surgery for brain tumors. She had been drinking lots of diet soda for years. There have been over ninety different reactions reported to the FDA for aspartame alone. I have read studies that show aspartame can break down into formaldehyde in the body. I ask my patients to quit using artificial sweeteners and see how much better they feel in a few weeks.

Sweet is one of the five flavors in Oriental cooking, but again they use everything in moderation. We need to break the sweet habit. There are four other delicious flavors in our foods (see the section on flavors of foods). One more thought, if diet sodas and sugar-free desserts really work, why is there so much obesity in America?

Sugar

Americans eat 20 percent more sugar now than in 1970. That is 155 pounds of sugar a year. Popular coffee drinks can have 300 to 600 calories; most of them are sugar. A double scoop of ice cream can have eleven teaspoons of sugar. A popular sundae has twenty-seven teaspoons. A can of soda has ten teaspoons. A cookie has one teaspoon of sugar. To convince yourself and your children, add ten teaspoons of sugar one at a time to a glass—no one would ever sit down to eat ten teaspoons of sugar! So why drink a soda?

Fruit juice is high in sugar, and I don't recommend it for children. Why start them on a sweet habit? If you only give them water, they will want water. Set an excellent example for them and drink water not soda.

Fructose is still sugar, and that is why I limit my patients' fruit servings to two a day. Vegetable juice is better for us than fruit. There are four to eight apples in a glass of juice. How many people would eat that many apples a day? If you did, you would get so much fiber you'd be full! Again, we must re-train ourselves to see what really is important is life. Does drinking a can of soda give you the same pleasure as playing with your kids or walking through your yard?

Natural sweeteners exist such as agave nectar, fruits, honey, real maple syrup, molasses, and stevia. Except for two servings of fruit a day, try to only use one serving a day of the other sweeteners.

Processed Food

Food processing is important, but unfortunately, it can sometimes border on food poisoning. Mother Nature has done a wonderful job for millions of years growing food, but humankind sure is messing it up. Not all of us can grow all the food we need, but we can grow a little tomato plant, some cucumbers, and peppers. It is wise to be concerned about the pesticides on our produce. The vegetables and fruit with the most residue are apples, celery, cherries, grapes, lettuce, peaches, pears, peppers, potatoes, spinach, and strawberries. Wash these off extremely well or buy organic produce. Local produce uses less pesticide than larger "farms." Lettuce is easy to grow, and with homegrown lettuce, you have the beginning of a safer salad. Processed food is loaded with chemicals that most people cannot pronounce. I encourage people to shop in the perimeter aisles of the grocery store, which is where the meats, fish, eggs, dairy, vegetables, and fruits are located.

How to Read a Label

If you buy foods with labels, you need to understand how to read one. It's easier than in the past but still very difficult. The FDA does a decent job making sure companies do not make misleading claims. Last year the FDA stopped a popular cereal company from stating that their cereal lowered cholesterol. In 2010, the FDA worked hard to continue this task. A lawsuit filed in California cited a number of fish-oil-supplement suppliers for selling products with high levels of PCBs. This type of situation is not new to the industry. The companies that my office uses were not named in the lawsuit.

However, I have stopped prescribing certain supplements because the company could not prove to my satisfaction that what was on the label was in the bottle or because I was not happy with the choice of fillers. Patients bring in their vitamins, and I show them how to read a label. We are all horrified with some of the ingredients listed such as sodium laureth sulfate or propylene glycol—components of antifreeze and cancer-causing sudsing agents. Why would that be in your vitamins? These products were not "cheap" either.

Be careful of so-called, nutritious packaged foods. When they state, it is whole grain, it is usually whole WHITE flour or refined flour. Some whole-grain muffin mixes contain five teaspoons of sugar for each muffin. If you made the muffin from scratch, it would have much less sugar. If it says high-fructose corn syrup, beware. And high-fructose corn syrup is in everything! Avoid artificial flavors—what's wrong with real flavors? Stay away from all trans fats. (See the section on fats.)

When you look at a label, it should be easy to see the calories. Reducing calories reduces weight. The fat content listed on the label comes next. Keep in mind that polyunsaturated and mono-saturated fats are good. Trans fat and saturated fat are not good. Also, how much sodium does this food have? The average person should not have more that 1500-2000 milligrams of sodium a day. We typically eat 3000 at least.

How much fiber is in this product? Remember, we need twenty-five to thirty grams of fiber a day. Companies now put the amount of sugar on the label under the carbohydrates. The less sugar, the better. Some cereals have as much sugar as a slice of chocolate cake. (Forget it!) Then comes the protein. We need about two grams of protein for every half pound of body weight (this is just a general guide because every person is different).

A popular dessert has 350 calories, 53 grams of carbohydrates, 4 grams of proteins, and 36 grams of sugar. I wouldn't eat it! This is 1/14 of a cake without icing. Let me try to explain how the Chinese eat. Other Asian countries have similar diets, but it's easier for me to find facts from the Chinese. Their diet works but may take some getting use to. I've also purposely eliminated foods that Westerns might consider "strange." Please read this section and keep an open mind. Thousands of years of feeding millions of people can't be all wrong.

The Best Diet

Confusion abounds as to what we should eat. As you can see, not everybody can eat everything. Unless we advise you not to eat something, you can help build health by incorporating more vegetables and fruits in your diet. Whole grains are good (oats, buckwheat, brown rice, rye, wheat, or quinoa) but on a limited basis.

Quinoa is a seed that is amino-acid compete, high in protein, manganese, magnesium, iron, copper, and phosphorus. It is low in calories and high in fiber. It is high in copper and manganese, which serve as co-factors for SOD enzyme. This delicious food can be used in place of grains in salads, soups, or just by itself. It has a nutty flavor and comes from Peru, Chile, and Bolivia where it's been a staple for over 5000 years. It makes a super "cereal"; just add milk and a little honey.

To find recipes using quinoa, you can simply search the Internet. It is available in health food stores and is inexpensive. Always rinse it off first or it will taste bitter. Add boiling water, cover, and simmer for fifteen minutes. Check to see if it needs more water. It is wheat free and has a low-gluten content.

Chicken is good for most people; beef is better for others. A qualified nutritionist (we have two on our staff) can help you determine a daily plan that is best for you. We recommend eating fish twice a week. Unfortunately, we need to carefully examine the source of our fish. I prefer wild not farmed. I like things more natural, and keeping fish in big tanks feeding them food just doesn't seem right to me.

Eating seven servings of vegetables a day with two servings of fruit is a prescription for excellent health. We also need oils and fats—the good ones. Certainly, any processed food is bad for us. Studies show that the average American eats out four times a week. If you have the "perfect diet" for the other seventeen meals, you might be able to handle the processed, over-salted, and fatty foods.

Your body is a magnificent machine. Its purpose all day and night is to keep you alive and healthy. Our bodies have the right tools to do this, but sometimes things go haywire, and there is a breakdown in health. Acupuncture, nutrition, a correct diet, exercise, breathing techniques, and AcuSET will help you obtain a better level of health—no matter how poor your health is at the start of your treatments. We have done it for thousands of people—now it's your turn!

Chapter 8

Oriental Nutrition

During the Tang Dynasty (618-907 AD), the Chinese doctor Sun Si-miao said that regulating a sick person's diet and lifestyle could fix most situations. If it didn't, then it was time to see the doctor for acupuncture and herbal medicine.

The Five Energies of Food

Another important aspect of nutrition is the Five Energies of Food. My favorite books on the subject are *The Chinese System of Food Cures* and *Chinese Natural Cures* by Henry C. Lu. Have you ever wondered why some people drank hot tea and felt better, and some drank it and didn't feel any better? It's because the energy of foods and beverages can create different sensations in the body. The five energies of food are cold, cool, neutral, warm, and hot. These energies do not refer to the temperature of the food but rather its energetic qualities.

We all understand that ice is cold and boiling water is hot. However, the temperature is only a temporary condition. After you drink ice water, it warms up in your stomach; after you drink a piping hot cup of coffee, it cools down to about 102 degrees in your stomach. What happens after the food is in your stomach makes the real difference. The stomach's job is to receive food and liquid and to cook them (the term is "rotten and ripen"). The stomach is the "pot on a fire." The Spleen Meridian takes the "pure stuff" and helps create the Qi for other meridians and organs. If you eat raw or cold foods (cold in temperature), it's harder for the stomach to cook them. When someone is sick, we tend to feed him or her soup. In winter, we tend to eat more soups and stews. These foods are easier to digest, using less Qi for the process.

Asians don't drink as many iced or cold drinks as we do in the United States. Starting a meal with a cold drink sets us up for digestive problems. It would be better to drink a warm drink as this would start to make a soup in your stomach.

Juices are also not the best thing to drink. A hundred years ago, people ate an apple or two a day. They did not juice eight apples for one glass of juice. We did not have refrigerated trucks to transport juice all over the country. People in Florida did not have access to the amount of apples they do today, and those in Ohio did not have an abundance of oranges. People ate the foods that grew in their area. Their bodies adapted to what was around them. Raw fruits tend to be dampening and can cause phlegm.

If you have a type of arthritis that causes your joints to feel hot, you are restless and perhaps irritable. You have intense stabbing pain. In that case, you would want to eat foods that are cooler to neutral in energy. If you have skin rashes that worsen with heat, you would want to eat cool foods to lessen your heat. On the other hand, if you had been caught in the rain in January and felt cold, you would do better if you had a cup of hot coffee or ginger tea. Why not a cup of hot tea? Tea is cold in nature. Ginger tea and coffee have a warm energy.

To determine what foods to eat, you need to know if you have a hot or cold constitution. Your acupuncture physician will determine that in your initial consultation and diagnosis.

A hangover in most cases can be treated with cold foods. People with weight problems tend to have meridians on the cool to cold side. Here is a list of energetic properties and common foods in which they are found.

COLD: bananas, bamboo shoots, clams, crabs, dandelion leaf, grapefruit, hops, kelp, lemon/limes, mangoes, mung bean sprouts, persimmon, rhubarb, salt, star fruit (carambola), seaweed, sugar cane, tomatoes, water chestnuts, watermelon, wheat germ, and yogurt.

COOL: amaranth, apple, artichoke, avocado, barley, bean curd (tofu), beer, black currants, blueberries, buckwheat, cauliflower, celery, chamomile tea, chrysanthemum tea, chicory, chicken egg whites, cranberries, cucumber, daikon (radish), duck eggs, eggplants, kelp, kiwi, lemon balm tea, lettuce, mandarin oranges, mangoes, marjoram (spice), millet, mint, mung beans, mushrooms (button), oranges, pears, peppermint, rabbit, radish, raspberry tea, sesame oil, soy sauce, spinach, strawberry, Swiss chard, tangerine, tea (black), wheat, wheat bran, and wild rice.

NEUTRAL: adzuki beans, alfalfa sprouts, almonds, apricots, beef, beets, black sesame seeds, broad beans, chickpeas,

Chinese cabbage, carrot, chicken egg yolk, corn, duck, fig, flax, goose, grapes, hazelnuts, herring, honey, lentils, licorice, liver (beef), kidney beans, cow's milk, human milk, olives, oysters, papaya, peas, peanuts, pineapple, pistachios, pomegranate, plum, pork, potato, pumpkin and pumpkin seeds, quail, raspberries, rice, saffron, salmon, sardines, sesame seeds, shark, string beans, sunflower seeds, sweet potatoes, turnips, whitefish, white sugar, yams, and yellow and black soybeans.

WARM: anchovy, anise seeds, basil, bay, blackberries, black beans, butter, capers, cardamom, caraway, cherries, chestnuts, chicken, chives, cinnamon, coffee, cloves, coconut, dates, dill, fennel, garlic, ginger, ginseng, green onion leaf, green onions, guava, (fresh) ham, jasmine tea, kale, leeks, liver (chicken or pork), lobster, goat milk, molasses, mussel, mustard leaf, nutmeg, oats, oregano, parsley, parsnips, peaches, quinoa, raspberries, rosemary, rye, sage, shrimp, spearmint, spelt, squash, sweet basil, sweet potato, turkey, thyme, turmeric, vinegar, walnut, watercress, and wine. Asparagus is considered slightly warm.

HOT: liquor, black pepper, cinnamon bark, cottonseed oil, horseradish, chili peppers, cayenne, lamb, trout, mustard, soybean oil, green pepper, red pepper, white pepper, and dried ginger.

The Five Flavors of Food

Foods have five flavors: pungent, salty, sour, bitter, and sweet. Some foods such as grapes can have two flavors (sweet and pungent). In the beginning of this book, we described the meridians and their properties. Each meridian has its own sound, time of day, color, body system, odor, emotion, and flavor. The Lung Meridian has the pungent flavors, Spleen has sweet, Kidney has salt, Liver has sour, and Heart has bitter. These flavors can be used to treat conditions of the body.

For example, the sweet flavor affects the Stomach and Spleen Meridians. We tend to eat many sweet foods in the United States and be overweight. The Spleen and Stomach Meridians work with digestion. In Western terms, we agree that sweet foods have more calories and therefore weight gain occurs. Sour foods can induce perspiration and are good when someone has a cold (ginger tea).

In Chinese cooking, all five flavors are used. They know that we all need a little of all flavors—again, balance in all things. The most familiar Chinese sauce in Chinese cooking contains a five-flavor spice with all five flavors. It is very subtle and can help balance your foods.

PUNGENT: black pepper, chive, cinnamon, cottonseed, dill, fennel, garlic, green onion, green pepper, marjoram, nutmeg, peppermint, radish, red pepper, rosemary, soybean oil, spearmint, sweet basil, white pepper, and wine. Slightly pungent are asparagus and caraway.

SALTY: artichoke, barley, clams, crab, human milk, millet, oysters, pork, salt, and seaweed.

SOUR: apple, apricot, grape, grapefruit, kiwi, mandarin orange, mango, olives, peaches, pineapple, plum, raspberry, strawberry, star fruit, tangerine, tomato, and vinegar. Extremely sour fruits are lemon, pear, and sour plum.

BITTER: asparagus, celery, chocolate, coffee, hops, lettuce, vinegar, wine, ginseng, and pumpkin. Slightly bitter are kidney beans and sunflower seeds.

SWEET: apples, apricot, bamboo shoots, bananas, barley, bean curd, beef, beets, black sesame seeds, black soybeans, Chinese cabbage, clams, coconut, coffee, corn, cucumber, dates, duck, eggplant, figs, ginseng, grapes, grapefruits, guava, honey, kidney beans, kiwi, malt, mandarin oranges, mango, cow's milk, human milk, mung beans, olives, oysters, papaya, peach, peanuts, pears, persimmon, pineapple, plum, pork, pumpkin, raspberry, potato, radish, adzuki beans, rice, saffron, sesame oil, shrimp, soybean oil, spearmint, spinach, squash, star fruit, strawberry, string beans, sugar cane, sunflower seeds, sweet potato, tangerines, tomatoes, walnuts, water chestnut, watermelon, wheat, white sugar, wine, and yellow soybeans.

Chocolate is bitter, so we add sugar and oils to it to make candy. These additives are dampening and can cause problems. Cola drinks are made with herbs and spices and can help digestion. But we add sugar water and drink them cold, which overwhelms the Spleen Meridian.

Corn can be good to eat as it has a neutral temperature. But because it is neutral and sweet, it can also become dampening if you eat it too often. Corn is the most popular vegetable in America and is used in many processed foods. *Read labels!* As you read the list of foods, it is easy to see why this country is in bad shape concerning health.

On the other hand, eggs are good to eat and easy to digest. Remember how your mom gave you a soft-boiled egg when you were sick? Coffee is in the bitter, pungent, and warm categories. It takes Yin and transforms it into a type of Qi. As the Qi moves outward, you feel increased energy. It can move stuck Qi, and this is good. On the other hand, if you don't make enough Qi from eating and sleeping, you can feel more of this boost from coffee. People drink coffee when they are tired, which creates a bad cycle.

Have you ever wondered why drinking coffee sometimes gives you loose stools? Coffee is warm and causes the stomach to heat up, causing loose stools. It is also a diuretic and causes us to urinate more. Urination also loses Qi. Therefore, coffee is only for the hardy, healthy person. Some people find it hard to quit drinking coffee, so we advise them to mix regular coffee with decaffeinated coffee to ease their way out. However, there are also issues with decaffeinated coffee so feel free to ask us for recommendations.

The Movement of Food

The essence of foods also moves in different directions in the body, according to the Asians. Qi moves up, down, and sideways. Lung Qi moves one way, and Stomach Qi moves another way. If Stomach Qi moves up, we vomit. If Lung Qi moves up, we cough. If the Liver Qi moves up, we get headaches. Triple Burner Qi needs to move down to keep the bladder and bowels working right.

This concept is a bit hard to understand, but you can still get it! Foods that move upward are good to eat in the springtime, for example, beets, apricots, beef, Chinese cabbage, carrots, celery, chicken egg yolks, duck, fig, grapes, mandarin oranges, kidney beans, olives, oysters, potatoes, pineapple, string beans, adzuki beans, mushrooms, rice, and yellow soybean.

Foods that move outward are good to eat in the summer and are hot in nature. This heat helps us perspire and cool off. These foods include black pepper, cinnamon bark, dried ginger, green and red peppers, soybean oil, and white pepper.

We need to eat foods that move downward in the autumn. These foods also help with asthma, vomiting, and hiccups, which are a reverse flow of Qi. These foods also tend to be cold, cool, or warm and are sweet and sour. They include apples, bamboo shoots, bananas, barley, tofu, chicken egg whites, cucumber, eggplant, grapefruit, lettuce, mung beans, peaches, persimmons, spinach, star fruit, strawberries, tangerines, water chestnuts, and wheat.

Foods that move inward and are good in the winter are clams, crabs, hops, kelp, lettuce, salt, and seaweed. These foods are bitter or salty in flavor.

Common Meridian-Related Foods

If you have problems with a particular organ, try to incorporate some of the foods recommended below:

Lungs: carrots, cinnamon twig, coriander, duck, garlic, ginger, ginseng, grapes, green onions, honey, milk, olive, peanuts, pears, peppermint, persimmon, radishes, sweet basil, tangerines, walnuts, water chestnuts, and wine.

Large Intestine: tofu, black pepper, Chinese cabbage, corn, cucumbers, eggplant, figs, honey, lettuce, nutmeg, persimmon, salt, spinach, sweet basil, white pepper, and yellow soybean.

Bladder: cinnamon bark and twig, fennel, and watermelon.

Kidney: black sesame seeds, caraway, chestnuts, chicken egg yolk, clams, dill seeds, plums, pork, string beans, tangerines, walnuts, and wheat.

Liver: black sesame seed, celery, chive, clams, crab, peppermint, plums, saffron, sour plums, vinegar, and wine.

Gallbladder: chicory.

Heart: chicken egg yolks, cinnamon twig, green peppers, milk, mung beans, persimmon, red peppers, adzuki beans, saffron, watermelon, wheat, and wine.

Small Intestine: adzuki beans, salt, and spinach.

Spleen: barley, tofu, beef, carrots, chestnuts, chicken, cinnamon bark, clove, coriander, cucumbers, dates, dill seeds, eggplant, figs, garlic, ginger, ginseng, grapes, green peppers, honey, kiwi malt, nutmeg, peanuts, pork, red peppers, rice, squash, string beans, wheat, white sugar, and yellow soybeans. *We want to protect the stomach/spleen Meridians and organs; food is an important way to build Qi.*

Stomach: barley, tofu, beef, black pepper, Chinese cabbage, celery, chestnuts, chicken, chive, clams, clove, corn, crab, cucumbers, dates, green onions, ginger, kiwi, malt, milk, mung beans, olives, pears, pork, radishes, rice, salt, squash, sweet basil, tangerines, vinegar, water chestnuts, watermelon, wheat bran, white pepper, and wine.

Ailment-Specific Foods

If you have one of these problems, try adding some of the foods below to your diet.

Alcoholism—bananas and spinach

Asthma—pumpkin

Bleeding Gums—mangos, brushing with salt

Blood Deficiency—beef, chicken eggs, and spinach

Burns—apply potatoes (not on open sores); include cucumbers and barley in your diet

Canker Sores—watermelon and star fruit

"Cold" Arthritis Pain—cherries

Constipation—bananas, Chinese cabbage, honey, papayas, pears, walnuts, tomato, spinach, pork, and sweet potatoes (before bed)

Coughs—honey, lemons (for mucus), mangoes, peaches, pears, strawberries, peanuts (dry cough), walnuts, star fruit, carrots, asparagus, pumpkin, radishes, water chestnuts, sunflower seeds, sesame oil, black sesame seeds, duck, chicken eggs, pork, tangerines, mandarin oranges, and thyme (to relieve cough)

Diabetes—spinach, water chestnuts, green beans, sunflower seeds, beef, and chicken

Diarrhea—figs, pineapple, carrots, barley, adzuki beans, green beans, mung beans, rice, chicken, beef, chicken eggs, and pork

Edema—grapes, barley, adzuki beans, kidney beans, mung beans, beef, duck, saltwater clams, and seaweed

Excess Mucus—clams, pears, radishes, and seaweed

Excessive Perspiration—peaches

Eyes—cucumbers, tofu, water chestnuts, and chicken

Hangovers—strawberries and star fruit

Headaches—green onions and radishes

Hemorrhoids—bananas, spinach, and saltwater clams

Hoarseness—strawberries and chicken eggs

Hypertension—bananas, celery, clams, kelp, mung bean sprouts, sesame, peanut and corn oil, persimmons, and tomatoes

Impotence—walnuts and shrimp

Improve Appetite—green and red peppers and ham

Indigestion—apples, mangoes, lemons (not with ulcers), pears, pineapple, strawberries, star fruit, barley, and carrots

Induce Perspiration to Break a Fever—cinnamon, coriander, green onions, and rosemary

Kidney and Bladder Stones—star fruit and walnuts

Kidney Weakness—sweet potatoes and kidney beans,

Lack of Perspiration—peppers and star fruit

Low Blood Sugar—apples, nuts, eggs, and sunflower seeds

Lubricate Intestines, Ease Constipation—bananas, cow's milk, figs, peaches, soybean, walnuts, and watermelon

Lubricate Lungs—apples, apricots, mandarin oranges, peanuts, persimmon, and strawberries

Morning Sickness—apples and rice

Night Sweats—grapes

Nosebleeds—spinach

Pain—honey, spearmint, and squash

Poor Appetite—tomatoes, chicken, and fresh ham

Premature Ejaculation—sweet potatoes

Promote Digestion—apples, nutmeg, papayas, pineapples, plums, radishes, and tomatoes

Promote Urination—asparagus, barley, Chinese cabbage, carrots, coffee, cucumbers, grapes, hops, kidney beans, lettuce, mandarin oranges, mango, mung beans, onions, pineapples, plum, star fruit, water chestnuts, watermelon, lemon juice, and parsley

Relieve Diarrhea—sunflower seeds

Relieve Thirst—cucumbers, mangos, persimmon, pineapple, and tomatoes

Sinus Congestion—green onions, put salt on two or three lemon slices and eat them quickly.

Skin Rashes—mung beans

Soften Hardness (Cyst, Lump, Tumor)—clams, kelp, and seaweed

Sore Throat Pain—figs, lemons with honey, strawberries, watermelon, cucumbers, and chicken eggs

Stomachaches—papayas, peanuts, and chives

Stomach Weakness—sweet potatoes

Toothaches—star fruit

Urination—corn, grapes, pears, strawberries, watermelon, barley (difficult urination), celery, eggplants, chives (blood in the urine), raspberries, water chestnuts, green beans, walnuts, carrots (frequent urination), lettuce, and onions (diminished urination)

Vomiting—pineapple

Foods to Help Correct Symptoms

After your initial consultation, you will be given a diagnosis. Check below to add the appropriate foods to help resolve your problems:

Blood Deficiency needs a tonic to build blood up. Try adzuki beans, apricots, beef, beets, chicken eggs, dandelion leaf, dark leafy greens (mustard, turnips, beets, collards, and spinach), figs, grapes, kidney beans, parsley, sardines, and watercress.

Blood Stagnation causes pain. To help your body heal, eat chestnuts, chili peppers, chives, crab, mustard leaf, onions, peaches, and vinegar.

Cold conditions need warming, so see the warm foods listed above.

Dampness shows as edema or phlegm. To resolve it, eat adzuki beans, alfalfa, anchovy, barley, broad beans, celery, clams, corn, daikon radish, garlic, green onions, green tea, horseradish, jasmine tea, lettuce, mushrooms, mustard leaf, onions, parsley, pumpkin, radishes, seaweed, and turnips. **Eliminate** from your diet bananas, dairy, juices, pork, oranges, tomatoes, sugar, and wheat as they help to cause dampness.

Heat includes fevers, hot flashes, general feelings of heat, red face, nosebleeds, dark urine, and hot hands and feet. These conditions need cooling foods. See the list above.

Phlegm or Mucus can be helped with almonds, clams, daikon radish, garlic, grapefruit, licorice, marjoram, mushroom, mustard leaf and seeds, olives, onions, pears, black pepper, peppermint, persimmons, radishes, seaweed, shrimp, tea, walnut, and watercress.

Slice a lemon, put salt on it, and eat it quickly (only if you are not on a very restricted salt diet). Eat two or three slices two to three times a day. Salt dissolves phlegm, and lemons are astringent.

Qi, the most important aspect of our bodies, must always be replenished. Eat the following as often as possible: beef, chicken, cherries, coconuts, dates, figs, grapes, fresh ham, herrings, honey, lentils, licorice, molasses, oats, potatoes (sweet and small red), rice, squash, tofu, and yams.

To Move the Qi (stagnation causes pain) eat carrots, radishes with these herbs and spices—basil, caraway, cardamom, cayenne, chive, clove, coriander, dill, garlic, marjoram, and turmeric.

Yin Tonics: apples, asparagus, chicken eggs, clams, crab, duck, duck eggs, honey, kidney beans, lemon, mango, oyster, peas, pears, pineapples, pomegranate, pork, string beans, tofu, tomatoes, watermelon, and yams.

Yang Tonics: chestnuts, lamb, lobster, pistachio nuts, raspberries, shrimp, and walnuts. These herbs and spices also help build Yang Qi—basil, chives, cinnamon bark, chives, dill, garlic, rosemary, sage, and thyme.

Chapter 9

Medicines

Herbal Medicines

I am very concerned with the herbal use in America. It is estimated that 25 percent of the population uses herbal medicines, mostly purchased through the mail or the local grocery/drug store. I have studied herbal medicine for the last twenty-five years and understand how complicated it is. The herbal medicines used in my practice are the best quality available. When you purchase herbs, please be diligent in your research.

The problem with imported herbals purchased through the mail or over the Internet is very simple. We do not know what is really in the bottles. There have been instances of labels stating a fake manufacturer or listing herbs not in the bottles. I know that some of the herbals can contain heavy metal, drugs, or allergens. Counterfeit medicines in China kill thousands of people each year. It is not uncommon to purchase a product that does not have the correct herb inside. It could have a similar species or use a part of the herb that would not do what you expect it to do.

The companies we deal with keep a constant watch over all the herbals imported and warn us of any potential problems in the sales throughout America. They buy and process the correct herbs and are constantly monitored by the Food and Drug Administration.

Homeopathic Medicines

Samuel Hahnemann (1755-1843) is the founder of homeopathy. He was a German physician, chemist, and medical translator. He wanted to find a safer, gentler, more effective type of medicine. He admired the ancient idea of "like cures like." He took the two words from the Greek language for "similar" and "suffering" to describe his new health care system.

Homeopathic medicine is made from substances in nature. Many of the medicines today have been developed from minerals and/or plants. Dr. Hahnemann found a way to reduce the harmful side effects from medicines by diluting them into micro-doses.

Homeopathy is very safe and gentle for all chronic and acute problems. It is also inexpensive. It is practiced in most countries. In Europe, homeopathy is a popular form of health care. In fact, you can choose between allopathic or homeopathic medicine when you go to your doctor or pharmacy. In the United States, for the most part, only "alternative" practitioners use homeopathy.

This was not always so. At the beginning of the twentieth century, one in every five medical doctors was a homeopath. Over a hundred homeopathic hospitals and twenty homeopathic medical schools existed. Homeopathy is credited for saving countless lives during a nationwide flu epidemic. After changes in medicine early in the last century, the schools gradually closed. The demise was due to politics and allopathic doctors with the advent of the mass production of prescription drugs. Now, there is a resurgence and interest in homeopathy in the United States, and schools are opening again. In 1992, the National Institutes of Health appointed a group of health professionals to evaluate the validity of all alternative therapies, including homeopathy.

In this practice, we use a homeopathic company that has been in business for over fifty years and is used worldwide. Another popular branch of homeopathy is the Bach Flower Remedies and Rescue Remedy. We ask you to fill out a Bach Flower Remedy questionnaire at the beginning of your treatment. Bach Flowers helps to ease the emotional symptoms you may be experiencing.

Dr. Edward Bach (1886-1936) was a physician in England at the beginning of the last century. He was introduced to homeopathy in medical school. He noticed that certain emotional symptoms would appear with specific physical symptoms. After years of research, he developed thirty-eight different flower remedies to help his patients along with the very famous Rescue Remedy. After you complete your questionnaire, we will determine the correct flower essences to use as an adjunct to your treatment.

You will find many books on homeopathy in this book's bibliography, in bookstores, and at your local library. Information also is available on the Internet.

Allopathic (RX) Drugs

It is estimated that over 100,000 people die each year in America from complications of over-the-counter medicines and prescription drugs. For example, over twenty-five drugs can interact with grapefruit. Imagine that—a wonderful fruit made by nature and you can't eat it if you are on certain medications. Fats and proteins can affect the absorption of some medications. Medications also block the absorption of nutrients. Many drugs cannot be combined with alcohol. Garlic can cause anti-diabetic medicines to increase serum insulin levels. Do you know if the medicines (over the counter or prescriptions) that you use are affected by food?

The potential of a bad drug/herb interaction is rare when dealing with a qualified practitioner. We know which herbs are safe with which medications and make a constant study of this. I will never take you off your prescription medicines. That is between you and your medical doctor. But as your health improves, you may not need a medication or will need a lower dose. Again, you need to discuss this with both your medical doctor and acupuncture physician.

If we prescribe any herbal medicines, it will be with the knowledge and educational background of many years with ongoing study and research. Hundreds of safe and effective formulas exist to heal any health problem. But I must know what medicines you take and when you take them. If there are any changes during your treatment schedule, please tell us.

The most important thing to remember is to take your prescription medicines and your herbal medicines two hours apart. If you are not on prescription medicines, we have wonderful potent formulas in easy-to-digest tablets. These tablets would be a short-term herbal prescription, not a lifelong can't-live-without-it product. Remember—we are trying to correct your problem and let your body do the job it was intended to do!

Chapter 10

Lifestyle Changes

Shampoo, Toothpaste, and Makeup

Shampoo, toothpaste, and makeup contain many chemical items. We have blindly been using personal care products for years without worrying. What we don't know can kill us. What we wear can be licked off, swallowed, absorbed through our skin, slip into our eyes, or breathed into our lungs.

Almost all of the face and body products that I have used for the last five years are natural. My skin and hair are in great condition according to my stylist. My makeup colors last all day. I heard natural shampoos would not lather as much. I experimented with different products (there are many on the market, especially compared to ten years ago), and I was pleased with the amount of lather. Besides, who told us we need lots of suds anyway?

What are these products doing to our environment and water? I like products NOT tested on animals. If you search the Internet for homemade beauty products, you will find thousands of ideas. Also try using homemade or safer house-cleaning products. Everything you breathe, ingest, or touch affects you. Let's become more diligent in protecting our families and ourselves.

Harmony and Emotions

After eleven years of working with patients, I see and hear about many negative things people say or do to themselves. We are our own worst enemies. I am not a counselor or psychologist, but I do have common sense. I have made these mistakes in the past. I still do at times, but I notice it more quickly and change my thoughts. Here are some very simple ideas in treating yourself better, which will reduce your stress and ease your pain. Love yourself: It then is easier to love others.

In Oriental medicine, everything boils down to Yin and Yang—balance in all things all the time. Balance also affects attitude. Each acupuncture meridian has an emotion connected with it. The Lung and Large Intestine Meridians work with the emotions of grief, sorrow, and letting go. The Kidney and Bladder Meridians are connected with anxiety and fear. The Liver and Gallbladder Meridians have anger, depression, and courage. In parts of Asia, they use the phrase: "Big Gallbladder" for someone with tenacity and "moxy." The Heart and Small Intestines Meridians are involved with joy (or lack of joy) and mania. Lastly, the Stomach and Spleen Meridians deal with sympathy, compassion, worry, and over-thinking (rumination).

Ask someone if they talk to themselves and they will deny it. Except we do, a million times a day. Usually it's not nice; in fact, it can be downright hateful. We will talk to ourselves in ways we would never talk to our friends or family. Remember that "you" will be hanging around with you until death. Start by loving yourself more; go slowly as this concept is new for most people. Praise yourself. Don't worry; no one but you will know what's going on. Give yourself a break, and don't be so hard on yourself. Filter out those negative thoughts; you can dump them down the toilet at anytime.

In all things, we have choices. Each situation or problem has two sides. It can be positive or negative; it can have a variation of degrees of good or bad. Ask yourself if worrying about this problem can actually fix it. Schedule a time to sit down to think about your situation if you can't deal with it immediately. Take time to cool off and keep your head clear. Make a list of pros and cons. Put a timeline down: Can it be fixed this week, now, or next year? Can you do anything right now or do you need to wait until daybreak? Can someone else be a sounding board for you or give you advice?

Most problems are age-old problems just with some slight twists. In Jazzercise the other day, my friend Joyce told another woman to "not talk the problem into existence." In other words, don't make statements aloud or to yourself, pronouncing that something may happen. Don't plan on rain ruining your picnic. In all my years of working with positive thinking, I had never heard that phrase (Don't talk the problem into existence). It's wonderful, and I will always be grateful to Joyce for it!

Almost everyone is familiar with a to-do list. It's helpful to habitually write down a list of the top ten priorities for the next day. This exercise can keep you organized and enable time for play and exercise. Yes, include play and exercise in your top ten things to do, and when you complete a task, cross it off. This little act sends a message of accomplishment to your brain and is a positive reinforcement.

Anticipate your next day in a positive light. It is ok to daydream about tomorrow and your plans. If you are concerned about a possibly difficult interaction with someone else, plan it out the night before. See it being resolved to your satisfaction. Think about the fun things in your life, the happy things. Be excited about them. These actions reduce the stress hormone cortisol and create a boost in endorphins (the feel-good hormones).

Wake up in the morning excited about a new day! Be grateful you woke up. Be grateful for your life, family, pets, friends, job, car, house, and so on. Feeling gratitude also releases those feel-good chemicals in your body. It becomes easier to do this with practice. At first, if you think you have very little to be grateful for or happy about, find one thing that doesn't hurt or just think about how you woke up in a house. After a few days, you will feel better about yourself and see all the wonderful things and people in your life.

If you can't or don't want to deal with the problem now, try these tricks. Mentally put your problem in a basket and tie balloons to it. Watch it float away. If you need to, see a string tied to the basket so you can pull it back to you when you feel ready to tackle it. You'll be surprised how little your basket is; I know it sounds silly, but it does help!

1. FIND SOMETHING YOU LIKE TO DO

Everyday do something for an hour, a minute, or however long you have, but do something you like to do, something that makes YOU happy. You may have to think about this for a while: What could make you happy? Schedule it into your day or evening.

2. SING ALOUD and LISTEN to MUSIC

No one has to hear you. It's amazing how much happier you will feel after two songs. Singing can cause levels of infection-fighting antibodies to increase, so sing around sick people (or wait till you get in the car) to keep healthy.

We play music during your acupuncture treatments. Great care goes into picking the right music because of the psychology of music and emotions. Mozart can help you learn to focus. We choose music that does not remind you of anything. It is instrumental and can relax your pulses and you.

3. LOOK AROUND

Gaze at flowers or trees; research has shown looking around stimulates certain waves in your brain. Look at a color you like. Blue is especially calming to all age groups. Watch your pet sleeping or playing. Go through a photo album of your vacations or family reunions—anything that makes you smile.

4. SMELL SOMETHING PRETTY

Our sense of smell connects with our brains. Walking into the house after someone has baked a pie or turkey brings instant smiles! Lemon and peppermint are invigorating, while lavender is calming. Vanilla is popular with men, while women prefer baby powder.

5. CLEAR OUT CLUTTER

Clutter in any area of our lives is overwhelming. Our brains don't like clutter or chaos. Every night, clean out one drawer, clear off your desk, or rearrange a shelf in a closet. It will make you feel better. Clean out your purse or briefcase. Don't try to tackle the whole house at once, just little bits at a time. Give things away; someone somewhere will need your unwanted stuff, and you will feel much better with fewer things.

6. YAWN

That's right—yawn! Right now. Do you feel smarter? Yawning happens for a few reasons: tiredness or being in a stuffy room. When you yawn, oxygen rushes in and stimulates parts of your brain that work with memory. Yawning also causes some of your neurotransmitters to work better, causing a happier feeling.

7. GET IN THE LIGHT

We need to be in the sunlight in the morning and again in the evening. Without the sunlight, we don't produce enough melatonin (see the sleep section). Ten minutes before ten AM and after four PM is safe without sunscreen and glasses (unless you are under doctor's orders NOT to do this).

Laughter

As I started writing this book, I asked myself what section I wanted to write first. Would it be explaining acupuncture, needles, herbals, weight loss, or something else? I was slightly amazed that I chose laughter. Laughter is important. It exercises your liver, sends oxygen to the brain, reduces stress hormone levels, relaxes and exercises your muscles, and sends out the feel-good chemicals. Laughter can lower blood pressure. Smiling uses fewer muscles than frowning! Kids laugh hundreds of times a day, and some adults don't laugh once a day. Kids smile over four hundred times a day, and adults smile only fifteen times at the most.

In my practice, I get to smile a lot more than the average adult as each time I enter a patient's room I put on a smile, and I smile again at them when they leave. It's easy to smile at my patients, and it makes me feel good! Practice smiling at strangers; you will receive smiles back.

In my experience, if something upsets me in the morning before I leave for work, I feel tense. I try not to watch the news while getting ready for my day but will put on a comedy or listen to a funny CD. I try to smile as I drive to work; people really can see into your car, and I find many others smiling back. Studies over the last twenty years have linked the effect of our emotions on our health or lack of it. I have noticed my most positive and happy patients do get better faster than the grumpy negative ones.

I understand how pain can make you feel miserable and not like smiling, so we work to lighten our patients' moods when they come in—even if by doing nothing more than just acknowledging that they feel miserable and hurt. We then try to give hope. There is always a laugh or a chuckle heard somewhere in our clinic through the day; we can't help it! People get well and that makes us happy! Laughing helps to relax muscles, and most pain causes muscles to tighten up. Laughing can help us see the situation in a different light: No matter how bad things are, they could be worse, so we laugh in gratitude!

Laughter can affect your attitude and that can affect everyone you meet. I receive jokes all day in emails from my family. I hope you do too. Enjoy them, take a minute to read them, and LAUGH aloud. Your pets like to hear you laugh also. Watch your pets for an easy way to stir up a chuckle! Laughter is free and easy to do. We all know how to do it, just sometimes we forget. You can't eat and laugh at the same time. Wouldn't it be fun to laugh every time you wanted to eat a cookie? And then not eat it! See, didn't that make you smile? You can spread happiness or anger. So smile at people in the grocery store or post office. It will lighten their heart and yours.

Laugh—you'll feel better!

Tension Releasers

A wonderful acupuncture point is located on your forehead between your eyebrows. It is called Yin Tang. You can tap it twenty times to relax.

Another point is on the inside of your arm three fingers up from your wrist in the middle. You can rub it for twenty seconds to relax.

To help with confusion or on days when you can't tell your right from your left, try this exercise. Make two fists and tap the pinkie sides together fifteen times.

Stretches

Never spend more than one hour at the computer without stretching. Stand up; reach up with both arms, palms facing each other. Bend forward as you inhale. When you bend forward as far as you can go, relax your hands and exhale. Inhale up with your hands facing each other and point to the sky.

Then let your arms hang loose and gently swing side to side. You can go faster and faster but don't lose your balance. Try to slowly work up to ten times on each side.

Now sit back down and slowly, very slowly, tilt your head to the right. Take a few seconds to do this. Raise your head back up and tilt to the left. Then drop your head forward again very slowly. Tilt your head back, very gently, and extend it back. Roll your shoulders gently back.

Take both hands and make opened fists (claw hands). Place your fingers on the top of your head (one on each side) and pull down to your ear—gently. Go down the sides and then do the back of your head.

Lastly, pretend you are swimming; raise your right arm and shoulder up and back and then do the same with your left side. Do this at least five times.

These stretches are good for children also. Always remember not to cradle your phone on your shoulder. Get a headset if possible.

Prayer/Meditation

Some people pray, some people meditate, and some don't do anything. Prayer and meditation are as old as people are. In the last ten years, research has shown that patients in a hospital who had prayers said for them improved faster than those who did not. Some skeptics challenge this, and we'll let them. Those of us that pray and meditate are happy to continue doing so. If at the very least you sit quietly on a daily basis for a few minutes and just express gratitude for waking up and experiencing life as you have it, you will feel better. There are thousands of book and CDs on prayer and meditation if you feel you need more instruction on expanding your practices. Try it again if you haven't in awhile. I truly recommend it.

Breathing Techniques

One of my favorite breathing techniques is to take a deep breath and fill my stomach with air so it pushes out. Then I hold to the count of four and slowly release the air, pulling my stomach against my backbone. You can play with this until you can do it with ease.

Work up to inhaling to a count of eight, holding for a count of eight, and releasing for a count of eight. Then try counts of sixteen or thirty-two. If you become dizzy, back down on the counts.

If you have a headache or sinus pressure, try this: Inhale deeply, push your stomach out. Hold for the count of four and exhale through your mouth. Do this fifteen times.

If you are tired, try this: Close your left nostril with your thumb and inhale through the right nostril for a count of four or eight. Move your thumb and close off the right nostril and exhale through the left nostril. Do these four to eight times.

The following is a breathing technique for the practice of Qi Gong. Sit or stand straight. Rest both hands below your belly button (it's ok to touch your body—it's yours). Breathe in and out through your nose. Exhale all the way out; when you think you are done, exhale a little more. Next, inhale all the way down to your belly, sticking out your belly when you do. Now you have more air in your lungs. Exhale all the way down. If you get dizzy (not breathing deeply in the past), sit down while you do this. Keep your chest relaxed during the breathing. See a small ball of light deep down in your belly; as you breathe, see it grow bigger and brighter. Do this "exercise" for eight inhales and exhales. During the day when you get stressed, do it at least for a minute. You'll notice an improvement in your mood and thinking.

For pain or anxiety, inhale through your nose for a count of four and exhale through your mouth for a count of four. Try to increase the count until you get to eight.

The last technique to help with stress is to inhale and hold it up to one minute. This takes practice but is well worth the effort.

Playtime

Exercise or "moving your body"—most people do not like to do it. But not exercising is not an option! We are composed of muscles, bones, tendons, and ligaments. They need to be active and strengthened on a daily basis. Exercise releases those feel-good chemicals. Studies show that weekly moderate exercise can decrease your weight and lower your risk of cardiovascular disease and cancer. Exercise also moves blood and nutrients to the brain.

Aerobic and weight-bearing exercise can decrease the risk of strokes and heart disease by 20 to 30 percent and of broken bones by 40 percent especially hips and spine and can lower the risk of diabetes by 30 to 40 percent. Additionally, it can aid in weight loss, can reduce the pain of arthritis, can lower blood pressure, and prevent depression (or help those who suffer with it). Other studies show older adults have a 30 percent lower risk of falls with walking, Tai Chi, and strength training.

Studies at a university in Missouri showed the most active people were 21 percent less likely to get colon cancer. Other studies have shown that moderate to vigorous exercise reduces the risk of breast cancer. These studies can be found through the Internet.

Weight gain is associated with a few cancers. The American Cancer Society recommends at least thirty minutes of moderate to vigorous activity five days a week. More would be better, but I am happy if my patients do that much. I remember a woman in her eighties that started working out at our gym before she went to Egypt. She wanted to be strong and agile enough to fulfill her lifelong dream of riding a camel. I watched her become stronger in less than six weeks. She was a thin woman to start with but with flabby arms, stomach, and butt. In six weeks, those body parts were firm; in fact, she had the derriere of a twenty year old when she left for her adventure. I loved seeing the picture she brought back of herself sitting atop a camel!

You're never too old to start working out in one form or another. A study from the University of Maryland showed people aged sixty-five to seventy-five who exercised three times a week for nine weeks showed an increase in muscle volume and could lift more weights. A nice side effect of weight training is that muscles fill in sagging skin, and we look younger.

Dieting without exercise produces slower results and even a brisk walk for thirty minutes a day can speed up weight loss. Exercise cleans out the lymphatic system, releases toxins through your sweat, and helps reduce stress. Strong muscles and ligaments reduce injury during falls and accidents. In my opinion, people who exercise regularly seem happier and more alive. Unfortunately, it seems that the people who need exercise the most are doing it the least.

As soon as you have an operation, the hospital staff has you up and moving as soon as possible. There is a reason for that. You lose calcium if you lie still in bed. Muscles atrophy, and Qi and Blood stagnate. There is always something you can do. If you are capable of exercising, pick something you like to do for fun. Walk around the mall if the heat is too much for you. Water aerobics is easy and safe, even for people with arthritis. You can find exercise shows on TV or rent or buy an exercise DVD.

Ballroom Dancing, Belly Dancing, Jazzercise and Zumba

Belly dancing or any type of dancing is fun and very helpful. My favorite exercise is Jazzercise. There are almost 18,000 instructors with over 32,000 classes a week. Jazzercise is fun, incorporates dance with stretching, increases your heart rate, and helps you feel graceful (well, not at first, you're too busy laughing at yourself). It is also inexpensive.

Zumba is another form of movement that is cardiovascular in nature. I swear there are times you know both feet are not touching the ground. You don't have time with jazzercise or Zumba to feel self-conscious, and no one else is watching you either; they're too busy having fun themselves.

If those two are too vigorous for you, try ballroom dancing. My husband and I did it for one and a half years, and we loved it. Here you do learn to be graceful. Our beloved instructor Bonnie had us proficient in at least one dance at the end of every class. I have a patient who manages a senior center, and she says the people who dance every week are healthier and go to the doctor less.

Play with your kids. We have a major obesity problem with children. Children spend more time in front of computers and playing videogames than outside. Walk your dog; she/he is probably overweight.

Some people can't stand up for long periods, so there are chair exercises that are easy to do. One is to hold a soup can in each hand, stretch your arms down to your sides, and slowly lift them to shoulder level. Start out with five times a day for one week.

At that point, you can increase the intensity by using two-pound weights or increasing the number of times you lift the soup cans. Walking around your house a three times a day will increase the Qi and Blood flow.

For healthier people, get to a class, work out at home, or go to the gym. Place that bike or treadmill you bought years ago (yes, the one the kids think is a clothes hanger) in front of the TV. Get on it every commercial and MOVE! If you have access to a swimming pool, do jumping jacks, run in place, bounce on one foot at a time, or walk across the shallow end for fifteen minutes at least. Hold on to the side of the pool and do leg lifts or kicks. Get up to your neck in water and pretend you are swimming with your arms. There are inexpensive weights and barbells to use in the pool. They work beautifully and have been a favorite of mine for years. If you can swim, do that; it's one of the best exercises for every area of your body. The opposing movement of your arms and legs not only helps your physical body but also your brain.

You can lie down on a bed or sit in a chair. Move your right hand across your body to your left knee as you raise that knee and touch the top of your knee. Repeat with your left hand. Alternate and do this for three minutes. This will relax you and help you focus.

Cleaning house (I mean really cleaning house) can be an aerobic exercise. Pulling weeds and gardening is great too. I rarely see fat gardeners. At the very least, turn on music and dance around your house. Your pets will see how happy you are and will participate too.

Just get up and do SOMETHING. Your health depends on it. Remember that people live to a ripe old age now. Do you want to be sickly and on lots of medicines or do you want to be healthy and active? The choice is really yours.

Tai Chi

Tai Chi is an ancient gentle form of exercise from China. Little children and the elderly practice it daily. It is very fluid, graceful, pretty to watch, and soothing to do. In Tai Chi, you breathe deeply with controlled movements. It keeps you in balance and helps with your balance. Having good balance prevents falls. A 2006 survey involving 6000 hospitals across the county showed that 47 percent of the hospitals offered Tai Chi or Qi Gong.

Qi Gong

Qi Gong is another form of controlled fluid movements with a little more action. It is effective in relieving stress and brings your body systems back to balance. Your goal in Qi Gong is to become "centered" in your body and mind.

During Qi Gong, you take deep breaths and exhale fully. This is relaxing, reduces stress, and can eliminate cravings. (See the section on Breathing.)

To help your eyes, rub your palms together to create some heat and place your hands over your eyes for five seconds. Repeat three times. Then gently press your thumb along the rim of your eyebrow from the inside to the outside (eyes closed) and above your eye socket. Use your ring finger and trace your eye (move from the outside of your eye to the inside gently).

The last eye exercise is to look to the right, then to the left, up, down, diagonal, and back to center. Do this up to five times. If this causes pain, STOP.

You can find Qi Gong DVDs and even instructional programs on most cable stations. No equipment is involved, and you can be in poor physical shape when you start.

Yoga

Throughout the world, people of ALL beliefs and religions practice yoga for stress relief, high blood pressure, flexibility, and strengthening muscle. The thousands-of-years-old program came from India. You do not have to "belong" to a religion to do yoga. It is not a religion. I have used yoga for flexibility and stress relief for over twenty-five years. I have always enjoyed it; we have incredible teachers locally as I am sure there are everywhere. In five minutes of the stretching and breathing, you can be very relaxed. In fact, some of the positions (called poses) need concentration, and you can't think of your problems. It's like a mini-vacation from life.

Neurotransmitters Testing

A great weapon against anxiety, depression, weight loss, insomnia, ADD, ADHD, addictions, some types of memory loss, PMS, menopausal symptoms, fatigue, and behavior issues is neurotransmitter testing and then treatment with the correct amino acids and nutritional protocols. I could write a book on this subject! We have treated children that I actually saw walking on walls—children who can't rest or settle down. Although, these children are usually very bright and intelligent. The test is simple, and the results are astounding in some cases. The nervous system maintains a delicate balance. It can be thrown off by diet, infections, injury, stress, genetics, and toxins. If every one of my patients was tested for neurotransmitter imbalance, I believe we would more quickly solve their other conditions.

Sleep

Before electric lights were accessible, we went to sleep when it got dark and woke up when it got light. I'm sure there were sleepless nights then, but people were exhausted from a hard day's work of physical labor. Almost 50 percent of Americans have some sort of sleep problems on any given night. Most can't sleep due to worries, and not sleeping well prevents us from figuring out how to handle our problems. Twenty-five percent of adults report chronic sleep problems

Adults need an average of seven to nine hours of sleep. Children need more—from ten to twelve hours a night. Teenagers (who get the least amount) need ten hours a night. We sleep two hours less a night than we did one hundred years ago, one hour less than fifty years ago, and twenty minutes less than ten years ago.

Less sleep interferes with our memory, thinking and decision capabilities, immune system, weight loss, and attitude. Children are affected even more by inadequate sleep. Why don't people sleep or sleep well? First look at what you do in the evening. You may have all the lights on and sit in front of a computer and/or TV. You watch the news or violent TV shows or movies. You eat high-sugar and high-fat foods loaded with additives. Lying down after big meals or snacks is very hard on the digestion. Your brain and body want to do other things besides digest food during the night. Your body prefers to do other jobs, especially healing. More than one alcoholic drink acts as a stimulant, and even if you fall into a drunken stupor, you are getting poor sleep.

You don't settle down with a good book or cuddle with loved ones unless it's the dog. You go over all the bad things that happened during the day. You review what you didn't say or did say that made you unhappy. You worry about bills, jobs, your family, your health, the government, the weather, and the stock market—all of which you cannot fix in the present moment, if ever.

We see three types of sleep problems in our clinic daily. The first one is the pattern of not falling asleep when you want to, the second is waking up around three to five AM ready to get up and go, and the third is not sleeping due to pain.

The first step to remedying this is to stand outside for ten minutes in the morning without sunscreen and sunglasses. In the early evening, do it again. Look up at the sky and smile; feel grateful for your life. This action tells our pineal gland it's time to wake up and to go to sleep, when to make melatonin and when to slow it down. This is how our ancestors lived.

When you can't fall asleep when you want to (ten PM is a great time to do that), it is usually due to cortisol excess (a stress response to your life). Play with your pets; read a book to your children. Put together a picture puzzle or do crossword puzzles. Do something to quiet your mind. Turn the TV and computer off one hour before bedtime. Take a warm shower or bath, not hot. Put on some soothing music and curl up in bed with a book (though not an exciting one). When you get to bed, make sure the room is on the cool side with no fans blowing on you. Turn the clock away from you, preferably across the room. Keep it dark in your room. No work is allowed! Now close your eyes and look to the right and slowly to the left. Do this for a few minutes. This will calm your brain.

The late evening would be a great time to start that inspirational or self-help book you've kept next to your bed. We've all seen the TV commercial about excess cortisol and weight gain especially around the waist. The one thing you can do at home is support your blood sugar. Eat a light high-protein snack one hour before bed. This can be a piece of cheese, six nuts, a glass of milk (no cookies), or a hardboiled egg.

This snack is also a great idea for the person that wakes up between three to five AM. When the blood sugar drops, you may wake up from a nightmare or just wake up quickly thinking about ALL you have to do, and you're ready to go. Again we are dealing with blood sugar. In Oriental medicine, one to three AM is the Liver time, and the emotions dealing with the Liver Meridian are anger and frustration. The Heart Meridian works with insomnia also. Circle your wrists with your other thumb and index finger and gently rub around your wrist. This soft pressure will help you to feel calm and release your problems.

The patient with pain that can't sleep misses out on the perfect healing time. We heal when we sleep. Consequently, the first thing we do with acupuncture is to ease pain to promote sleep. We can also do this with homeopathic or herbal medicine. Calcium is a painkiller, and magnesium is a muscle relaxer; both will help you sleep. Some herbal teas on the grocery store shelves are calming too.

Chiropractic

Chiropractic care has a history as old and as rich as acupuncture. Twenty-two million people a year receive chiropractic manipulations in the United States. Doctors of chiropractic (also called chiropractors and chiropractic physicians) practice a drug-free, hands-on approach to establishing health in the body. Most people are familiar with chiropractic for back pain, although it is helpful in many more conditions. Chiropractic physicians must have a degree from a four-year accredited college in pre-med before they attend an accredited (by the US Department of Education) chiropractic college. They are required to finish 4200 hours of education and intern in a clinic also. They are licensed in all fifty states and have been for many years. Chiropractic is extremely safe. For more information, go to www.acatoday.org.

Massage

Massage is a healing art that is as old as acupuncture and chiropractic if not older. the first response to pain is to rub the area. Massage helps reduce stressful feelings, improves circulation, stimulates the flow of lymph (defense system) and just feels good! Massage therapists are educated and licensed. Give your massage therapist feedback during your treatment as some people like a gentle touch and others like more intense pressure. You can also massage yourself. It would not be the same as a professional, but it's your body; it is ok to touch it.

Tapping

Eleven years ago I came across a procedure called the Emotional Freedom Technique that sounded too good to be true. Since it worked with acupuncture points, I decided I needed to investigate; it really does work! I have continued to come across variations of it. I use it and instruct patients on the wonderful relief it can give. A close friend and Mental Health Therapist Lauren Griffin simplified the process and can teach anyone in an hour. The more you tap, the easier it is to do. A self-help protocol, you can do it in public, and no one will know you're doing it. I do it when I am in traffic for stress. Tapping is super for any pain. I hear some amazing feedback from patients who are "tapping."

Each day, each minute, each second we can make the choice to change something in our lives. To get started all we need is the "willingness" to take that next positive step. One less cookie, one less glass of wine, one less negative attack on yourself, one less "whatever." Be willing to plan your positive steps, set goals, write them down and review them during the day. Make that commitment to yourself to become healthy in all ways. It takes 21 one days to make or break a habit. You can make the decision to be willing to start and stay with your plan.

This book could have been over a thousand of pages; it boils down to a few simple guidelines. Please take at least one idea and change your life for the better.

Acupuncture is an incredible healing modality proving itself over and over for thousands of years. In the very near future I know it will be readily available to all who desire to take charge of their own health and realize that many of the "things" you have done in the past aren't working. Acupuncture treatments can help you sort out your next steps in changing your mind, attitude, and life as it works on the whole being, not just an ache or pain. Acupuncture brings balance to you, your Qi, Yin, Yang and Blood.

BREATHE MORE

EAT LESS

EXERCISE MORE

WORRY LESS

LOVE YOURSELF MORE!

Bibliography

Acupuncture: Everything You Ever Wanted To Know, Dr. Gary F. Fleischman, 1998, Barrytown Ltd., Barrytown, New York.

Acupuncture in the Treatment of Children, Julian Scott & Teresa Barlow, 1986, Eastland Press, Seattle, Wash.

Applying Bach Flower Therapy to the Healing Profession of Homeopathy, Cornelia Richardson-Boedler, NMD, HMD, MA, MFCC, UKMHMA, 1998, B. Jain Publishers (P) Ltd., Paharganj, New Delhi, India

A Practical Dictionary of Chinese Medicine, Nigel Wiseman and Feng Ye, 1998, Paradigm Publications, Churchill Livingstone, London, England.

A Practitioner's Guide to Herb-Drug Interactions and Safety, Andrew Gaeddert, 2007, Oakland, California (study guide from Health Concerns).

Anti-Aging Manual, Joseph B. Marion, Information Pioneers Publishing, Woodstock, Conn.

Art of Palpatory Diagnosis in Oriental Medicine, Skya Gardner-Abbate, 2001, Churchill Livingstone, London, England.

Between Heaven and Earth, Harriet Beinfield, L.Ac. and Efrem Korngold, l. Ac., O.M.D. 1991, Ballentine Books, New York, New York.

Biochemical, Physiological, Molecular Aspects of Human Nutrition, Martha H. Stipanuk, 2006, Saunders, St. Louis, Missouri.

Botanical Influences on Illness, Melvyn R. Werbach M.D., Michael T. Murray N. D., 1998, Third Lane Press, Tarzana, California.

Breaking the Aging Code, Vincent C. Giampapa, M.D., F.A.C.S., and Miryam Ehrlich Williamson, 2004, Basic Health Publications, Bo. Bergen, N.J.

Change Your Brain, Change Your Life, Daniel G. Amen, M.D., 1998, Three Rivers Press, N.Y., N.Y.

Chinese Healing Secrets, Bill Schoenbart, L.Ac., 1998, Publications International Ltd. Lincolnwood, Il.

Chinese Natural Cures, Henry C. Lu, 1986, 1990, 1991, 1994, Black Dog and Leventhal Publishers, New York, New York.

Chinese Pulse Diagnosis, Leon I. Hammer M.D., 2005, Eastland Press, Seattle, Washington.

Chinese System of Food Cures, Henry C. Lu, 1986, Sterling Publishing, New York, New York.

Clinical Applications of Ayurvedic and Chinese Herbs, Kerry Bone, 2000, Phytotherapy Press, Queenland Australia.

Clinical Guide to Nutrition & Dietary Supplements in Disease Management, Jennifer Jamison, MBBCh, PhD, EdD, FACNEM, Grad Dip Human Nutrition, Professor of Diagnostic Sciences, RMIT University Victoria, Australia, 2003, Churchill Livingstone, London, England.

Cupping Therapy, Ilkay Zihni Chirali, 1999, Harcourt Brace and Company, London, England.

DeGowin's Diagnostic Examination, Richard L. DeGowin, M.D., FACP and Donald D. Brown, MD, FACP, 2000, McGraw-Hill, New York, New York.

Detoxify or Die, Sherry A. Rogers, M.D., 2002, Sand Key Company, Sarasota, Florida.

Dr. Chi's Method of Fingernail and Tongue Analysis, Tsu-Tsair Chi N.M.D., Ph.D., 2002, Chi's Enterprise.

Drugs That Don't Work and Natural Therapies That Do, David Brownstein, M.D., 2009, Medical Alternative Press, West Bloominfield Mich.

Electromagnetic Fields, B. Blake Levitt, 1995, Hartcourt Brace, Orlando, Florida.

Fight for Your Health, Byron J. Richards, 2006, Wellness Resources Books, Minneapolis, Mn.

Fluid Physiology and Pathology in Traditional Chinese Medicine, Steven Clavey, 1995, Churchill Livingstone, London, England.

Fundamentals of Chinese Medicine, Nigel Wiseman, Andrew Ellis, and Paul Zmiewski, 1985, Paradigm Publications, Brookline, Massachusetts.

Fundamentals of Clinical Nutrition, Sarah L. Morgan and Ronald L. Weinsier, 1998, Mosby, St. Louis, Missouri.

Golden Needle, Wang le-Ting, Yu Hui-chan & Han Fu-ru, 1996, Blue Poppy Press, Boulder, Co.

Gua Sha, Arya Nielsen, 1995, Churchill Livingstone. New York, New York.

Heart Sense for Women, Stephen T. Sinatra, M.D., 2000, Lifeline Press, Washington, D.C.

Homeopathic Medicine at Home, Maesimund B. Panos, M.D. and Jane Heimlich, 1980, G. P. Putnam's Sons, New York, New York.

Homeopathic Self-Care, Robert Ullman, N. D. and Judith Reichenberg-Ullman, N. D. 1997, Pima Publishing, Roseville, California.

Iodine, Why You Need It, Why You Can't Live Without It, David Brownstein, M.D. 2009, 4th Edition Medical Alternative Press, West Bloomfield, Mich.

Immunotics, Robert Roundtree, M.D., and Carol Colman, G.P., 2000, Putnams Sons, New York, New York.

Journal of Chinese Medicine Number 9, April 1982, *History of Acupuncture*, Giovanni Maciocia.

Journal of Chinese Medicine Number 21, May 1986, *A Brief Study of the History and Ancient Literature on Acumoxibustion*, Wang Xuetai.

Journal of Chinese Medicine Number 29, January 1989, *Outline of the History of Acupuncture in Europe*, Elisabeth Hsu.

Life: Conquest of Energy, Richard M. Tullar, 1972, Holt, Rinehart and Winston, New York, New York.

Live Free from Asthma and Allergies, Dr. Ellen Cutler, D.C., 2007, Celestial Arts, Berkeley, California

Manual of Dermatology in Chinese Medicine, Shen De-Hui, Wu Xin Fen, Nissi Wang, 1995, Eastland Press, Seattle, Washington.

Micro Miracles, Dr. Ellen Cutler, D.C., 2006, Rodale Press, Emmaus, Pennsylvania.

Natural Answers for Women's Health Questions, D. Lindsey Berkson, 2002, Fireside Simon & Schuster New York, New York.

Neurology for the Non-Neurologist, William J. Weiner & Christopher G. G1989oetz, J.B. Lippincott Company Phil., Pa.

New Choices in Natural Healing, Prevention Magazine Health Books, 1995, Rodale Press, Emmaus, Pa.

Nutritional Support of Medical Practice, Howard A. Schneider, Carl E. Anderson, David B. Coursin, 1977, Harper & Row, Philadelphia, Pennsylvania.

Optimal Wellness, Ralph Golan, M.D., 1995, Ballantine Books, New York, New York.

Overcoming Thyroid Disorders, David Brownstein, M.D., 2002, Medical Alternative Press, West Bloomfield, Mi.

Physicians' Desk Reference for Herbal Medicines, 1998.

Perspectives in Nutrition, Wardlaw, Hampl, and DiSilvestro, 2004, McGraw Hill, New York, New York.

Pharmacodynamic Basis of Herbal Medicine, Manuchair Ebadi, 2000, CRC Press.

Please Don't Eat the Wallpaper, Dr. Nancy Irven, 2008, Morgan-James Publishing, LLC, Garden City, NY.

Practical Diagnosis in Traditional Chinese Medicine, Tietao Deng, 1991, Churchill Livingstone. London, England.

Principles and Practice of Phytotherapy, Simon Mills and Kerry Bone, 2000, Churchill Livingstone, London, England.

Salt, Your Way to Health, David Brownstein, M. D., 2006, Medical Alternative Press, West Bloomfield, Mich.

Say Good-bye to ADD and ADHD, Dr. Devi Nambudripad, 1999, Delta Publishing Company, Buena Park, California.

Silent Spring, Rachael Carson, 1962 Houghton Mifflin Company, Boston, Mass.

SUPER HEALTH, 7 Golden Keys to Unlock Lifelong Vitality, KC Craichy, 2005, Bronze Bow Publishing.

The Acupuncture Response, Glenn S. Rothfeld, M.D., M. Ac., and Suzanne Levert, 2001, Contemporary Books, McGraw Hill. New York, New York.

The Art of Acupuncture Techniques, Robert Johns, 1996, North Atlantic Books, Berkley, Ca.

The Biology of Belief, Bruce H. Lipton, Ph.D., 2005, Mountain of Love/Elite Books, Santa Rosa, California.

The Body Electric, Robert O. Becker, M.D. and Gary Selden, 1985, William Morrow, New York, New York.

The Cholesterol Hoax, Sherry A. Rogers M.D., 2008, Sand Key Company, Sarasota, Fl.

The Coenzyme Q10 Phenomenon, Stephen T. Sinatra, M.D., F.A.C.C., 1998,

Lowell House, NTC/Contemporary Publishing Group, Los Angeles.

The Complete Book of Chinese Health and Healing, Daniel Reid, 1994, Shambhala Publications, Boston, Massachusetts.

The Complete Idiot's Guide to Acupuncture & Acupressure, David W. Sollars, L.Ac., 2000, Penguin Books, New York, New York.

The Complete & Up to Date Fat Book, Karen J. Bellerson, 1993, Avery Publishing, Garden City, New York.

The Foundations of Chinese Medicine, Giovanni Maciocia, 1989, Churchill Livingstone, London, England.

The Guide to Healthy Eating, David Brownstein, M.D. & Sheryl Shenfielt, C.N., 2006.

Healthy Living, The Merck Manual of Diagnosis and Therapy, 1992, Merck Research Laboratories, Birmingham, Mich.

The Metabolic Typing Diet, William Wolcott and Trish Fahey, 2000, Broadway Books, N.Y., N.Y.

The Mind & The Brain, Jeffrey M. Schwartz, M.D. and Sharon Begley, 2002,

Regan Books, an imprint of Harper Collins Publishers, N.Y., N.Y.

The New Nutrition, Dr. Michael Colgan, 1995, Apple Publishing, Rahway, New Jersey.

The Nutrition Desk Reference, Robert H. Garrison, Jr., M.A., R.Ph., and Elizabeth Somer, M. A., 1985, Keats Publishing, New Canaan, Connecticut.

The Secret of Chinese Pulse Diagnosis, Bob Flaws, 1995, Blue Poppy Press, Boulder, Colorado.

The Tao of Healthy Eating, Bob Flaws, 1997, Blue Poppy Press, Boulder, Colorado.

The Web That Has No Weaver, Ted J. Kaptchuk O.M.D., 1996, Congdon & Weeds, Chicago, Illinois.

The Yellow Emperor's Classic of Internal Medicine translated, with an introductory study by Ilza Veith, 1966, First University of California Press Edition, Berkeley, California.

Understanding Acupuncture, Stephen J. Birch and Robert L. Felt, 1999, Churchill Livingstone, London, England.

Wellness Against All Odds, Sherry A. Rogers, M.D., 1994, Prestige Publishing, Syracuse, N.Y.

What Your Doctor May Not Tell You About Hypertension, Mark Houston, M.D., Barry Fox Ph.D., Nadine Taylor, M.S., R.D., 2003,Warner Books, and N.Y., N.Y.

Why Do I Need Whole Food Supplements?, Lorrie Medford, C.N., 2006, LDN Publishing, Tulsa, Oklahoma.

Why Do I Really Need Herbs?, Lorrie Medford, C.N., 2004, LDN Publishing, Tulsa, Oklahoma.

Winning the War against Immune Disorders & Allergies, Ellen Cutler, D.C., 1998, Delmar Publishers, Albany, New York.

You Staying Young, Michael F. Roizen M.D., Mehmet C Oz, M.D., 2007, Free Press, Published by Simon & Schuster, N.Y., N.Y.

www.acufinder.com/articles, 2007, 2008, 2009, 2010.

www.accpuncturetoday.com/articles, 2007, 2008, 2009, 2010

Acupuncture Terms

Astringe: to dry dampness

Blood (Xue): The Oriental explanation of Blood differs from the Western explanation. In the Oriental philosophy, Blood is the densest fluid substance in the body; it is a form of Qi. Blood gives nourishment and supports our bodies. Blood moistens the skin, hair, tongue, eyes, and sinews. Blood helps to anchor the mind and calms the emotions. If someone can't sleep, we say the mind floats. Blood is stored by the Liver, generated by the Spleen, governed by the Heart, and is the mother of Qi.

Cold: Are you colder than the people around you? Cold problems are characterized by aversion to cold, desire for heat, hypoactivity, lack of thirst, loose stool, paleness, lethargy, dullness, weakness, large amounts of clear urine, thick odorless discharges or phlegm that is usually white in color, pain, cramps, and spasms. A Cold condition is treated differently from a Hot condition.

Damp Heat: This is a condition of dampness and heat that occurs in the Large Intestine (diarrhea with mucus and blood), Bladder (urinary tract infections, kidney stones), and Gallbladder (gallstones).

Dampness: Can also occur due to living in a damp house or a physical condition. Dampness in the body usually appears during damp and humid weather. Symptoms are feelings of heaviness in the head and limbs, swelling, bloating of chest and abdomen, edema, nodular masses, watery stool, sore joints, large amounts of sticky discharges, phlegm, and lethargy.

Deficiency: A lack of Qi or Blood or a result of the weakened function of the organs or meridians. Over time, a deficiency can develop physical and emotional symptoms and signs, which are considered "normal" health problems.

Deqi: Translates as "arriving of Qi"—the feeling of obtaining the Qi with the needle, which the patient may experience as a slight pressure, fullness, numbness, or a tingling sensation. These sensations are normal and let the acupuncture physician know that the treatment is working. This is the "product" of major research across the world since the early 1950s. Books written as early as AD 652 talk about Deqi.

Disharmony: Lack of harmony and balance in the body due to the stagnation or imbalance of Qi. This can be caused by physical or emotional trauma, environmental factors, or an excess or deficient condition.

Disperse. A needling technique that moves, circulates, and distributes Qi to relieve the stagnation of Qi and Blood, or the accumulation of Heat, Cold, Dampness, or Phlegm.

Distal Points. Acupuncture points that are away from the area of pain or disease. For example, we can use a point on the hand for a toothache rather than needling the cheek.

Dryness. Affects the fluids of the body. Symptoms may include dry skin, chapped lips, dry cough, dry mouth, dry eyes, and constipation.

Eight Principle Patterns. Signs and symptoms have a deeper meaning in Oriental medicine. We look at patterns to find the cause; this helps us to organize diagnostic information according to the principles of Yin, Yang, Interior, Exterior, Hot, Cold, Excess, and Deficiency.

Essence (Jing): The material basis of an individual's life. It starts with our parents. It is stored in our Kidneys and is fluid like Qi. It is very precious and must not be squandered by excess alcohol, sex, poor diet, overworking, lack of rest, or a wild lifestyle.

Excess: When Qi, Blood, phlegm, urine, sweat, and tears are out of balance and accumulate, leading to symptoms and signs of an abundant nature.

External Factor: External factors are Cold, Damp, Wind, Dryness, and Heat and can affect the body.

Food and Environmental Sensitivity Assessment: This is a computerized electrodermal screening that helps to identify your body's response to certain foods and items you may come in contact with. See chapter 5 for more information.

Heat: Illness caused by heat is demonstrated by constipation, dehydration, fever, hyperactivity, inflammation, swelling, skin rashes, restlessness, agitation, insomnia, scanty dark urine, and strange-smelling body secretions.

Holistic: The word comes from the Greek "holos," meaning whole. Holistic medicine involves all areas of your life. We don't just treat your indigestion, but all the other symptoms. We treat with a philosophy that includes a comprehensive and complete agenda to heal your mind and body through exercise, diet, acupuncture, chiropractic, reflexology, and massage.

Homeostasis: The ability of the body to maintain sameness. Homo means man, stasis means same. The body does this by adjusting physiological processes, despite constant varying external conditions.

Imbalance: Lack of balance that leads to stagnation, weakness, or excess of Qi and our internal environment. This will lead to illness, disease, and pain.

Internal Factors: Any factors affecting the body that comes from the inside of the body. This is usually due to an imbalance or disharmony of meridian and organ systems.

Meridians: Also called channels. These are pathways in which the vital energy called Qi circulates through the entire body. Meridians are connected to every organ system. There are fourteen main meridians and many other channels.

Meridian Stress Assessment: Computerized electrodermal screening programs that will help us determine the start of your meridians (pathways). It will show us which meridians are on the low side or high side pertaining to energy. You will get a printed computerized diagram. In addition, we will take your pulse measurements manually.

Organ Systems: The five organ systems—Liver/Gallbladder (Wood), Heart/Small Intestines (Fire), Spleen/Stomach (Earth), Lung/Large Intestines (Metal), and Kidney/Bladder (Water)—organize all physical and mental processes and join together all of the structural components of meridians, cells, tissues, muscles, and organs. Each organ system is connected to a meridian. Together, they do everything that needs to be performed in our bodies.

Pathogen: An external factor such as bacteria, virus, or fungus that can cause illness, disease, and pain.

Phlegm: Comes after dense, congealed dampness that can cause cysts, obstructions, mucus, nodules, lumps, or tumors. It can be yellow, white, red, clear, or brown.

Qi: The pictograph or Chinese character of Qi means "vapor," "steam," "gas," and uncooked "rice." It can be as immaterial as vapor or as material as rice.

Sedation: Two conditions of excess in the body under physical stress. An excess or a deficient condition. Excess must be calmed down, or "sedated," with needles or herbs.

Seven Emotions: Throughout life, we experience many different emotions, some more than others. When these emotions are repressed, hidden, erratic, or excess, it can lead to disease and illness. These emotions correspond with a meridian. The seven emotions are shock and joy (Heart); anger (Liver); fear (Kidney); sadness (Lung); and worry and pensiveness (Spleen/Stomach).

Spirit (Shen): Refers to the mind and emotions. How you view life and relate to others. We can see it in your face and your eyes and hear it in your voice and your speech.

Stagnation: Occurs when Qi and Blood don't move. It is pain or bruising.

Tonify: An acupuncture needling technique used to nourish, supplement, support, and invigorate your body through the meridians and Qi. To tonify is to add to the body's vital energies to restore and promote homeostasis of the organ systems.

Traditional Chinese Medicine (TCM): An ancient and complete holistic system of health care that has been around for more than three thousand years. It includes acupuncture, herbs, Oriental nutrition, movement, and balancing the Qi and Blood to bring the body back to homeostasis.

Wind: A Wind illness affects the lungs, throat, head, and skin and is demonstrated by aversion to drafts, spasms, pains that move from body part to body part (a key factor in diagnosing), dizziness, vertigo, trembling, itching, headache, stuffy nose, scratchy throat, and numbness. These symptoms occur suddenly. When you suffer from "the common cold," an acupuncture physician will diagnose it as Wind Heat with a sore throat and fever or Wind Cold without a sore throat but with sniffles, runny nose, and sneezing.

Yang: One of the two forces that organize the universe and all in it. Yang manifests as fire, heat, restlessness, dry, hard, daytime, sun, energy, expansion, light, time, activity, and male birth. See this chapter for more information.

Yang Organs: Known as the "hollow organs" that transform matter, transport and store body substances, and discharge waste. The Yang Organs are the Gallbladder, Small Intestine, Stomach, Large Intestine, and Urinary Bladder.

Yin: One of the two forces that organize the universe. Yin manifests as moon, shade, rest, earth, female, blood, solid, soft, darkness, quietness, cold, inertia, and death.

Yin Organs: Known as the "solid organs" that store the essences of the body. The Yin organs are the Liver, Heart, Spleen, Lung, and Kidney.

Index

Deafness
  acupuncture treatment for, 75
Deficiencies, 48
  in the Blood, foods in Oriental
    nutrition specific to, 145
  defined, 186
  one of the eight principle
    patterns, 187
Dental problems
  acupuncture treatment for, 69–70
Depression
  acupuncture treatment for, 70
Deqi, 35
  defined, 186
Detoxification, 41
Diabetes
  foods in Oriental nutrition
    specific to, 146
Diagnosing your problem, 21–24
  look, listen, smell, and touch, 21
  pulse diagnosis, 21–23
  tongue diagnosis, 23–24
Diarrhea. *See also* Bowel conditions
  foods in Oriental nutrition
    specific to, 146, 148
Diet. *See also* Weight loss
  best for good nutrition, 134–135
Digestion
  acupuncture treatment for
    problems with, 70–74
  foods in Oriental nutrition
    specific to promoting, 148
Disharmony
  defined, 186
Disperse
  defined, 186
Distal points, 82–83, 92
  defined, 186
Diverticulitis. *See* Bowel conditions

Dizziness, 9
  acupuncture treatment for, 74
Dr. Oz
  role in spreading word of
    acupuncture, 4
Dreams, 108
Dryness
  an external factor, 187
  defined, 187
Du (governing vessel) Meridian,
    15–16
Duke University, 9, 87
Dyspena
  in cancer patients, 9

E

E-coli infection, 60
Ear acupuncture
  latest research on, 13–14
Earache
  acupuncture treatment for, 75
Earth
  role in the Spleen/Stomach
    organ system, 188
Eating. *See also* Overeating;
    Weight loss
  in a relaxed setting, 74
Edema
  foods in Oriental nutrition
    specific to, 146
EDS test. *See* Electrodermal
    computerized screening test
Eight principle patterns, 187
  Cold, 187
  Deficiency, 187
  defined, 187
  Excess, 187
  Exterior, 187

F

Nutrition, *(cont.)*
    minerals, 115–121
    portion control, 129–130
    processed food, 131–132
    sugar, 130–131
    supplements, 99–105
    Vitamin A, 105–106
    Vitamin B Complex, 106–110
    Vitamin C, 111–112
    Vitamin D, 112–113
    Vitamin E, 114
    Vitamin K, 114
Nutritional assessment, 28

O

Odors in diagnosis, 11, 16, 21, 62
Office visits—beginning treatment, 25–33
    computerized meridian assessments, 29–30
    electrodermal computerized testing, 30–33
    missed appointments, 33
    nutritional assessment, 28
    our clinic, 27–28
OM. *See* Oriental Medicine
Omega-3 fatty acids, 126
Omega-6 fatty acids, 125
Opiods
    endogenous, 9
Oprah
    role in spreading word of acupuncture, 4
Oregon Health and Science University, 8
Organ systems, 188–189
    defined, 188–189
    described, 188–189

Organ systems, *(cont.)*
    Heart/Small Intestines (Fire), 188
    Kidney/Bladder (Water), 188
    Liver/Gallbladder (Wood), 188
    Lung/Large Intestines (Metal), 188
    Spleen/Stomach (Earth), 188
Oriental Medicine (OM), 7–20
    balance introduced, 17–18
    Blood introduced, 19–20
    latest research in, 8–17
    principles of, 11
    Qi introduced, 18–19
    Yin and Yang introduced, 20
Oriental nutrition, 137–150
    ailment-specific foods, 145–148
    common meridian-related foods, 144–145
    the five energies of food, 137–140
    the five flavors of food, 140–143
    foods to help correct symptoms, 149–150
    the movement of food, 143–144
Original Qi (inherited), 18
Osteoarthritis, 51
Osteomalacia, 112
Overeating, 94–95, 102. *See also* Portion control
Oz, Dr.
    role in spreading word of acupuncture, 4

P

Pain
    foods in Oriental nutrition specific to, 147
    reducing, 10, 49–52
    treating postoperative, 9

www.acudebra.com